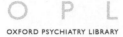

OXFORD PSYCHIATRY LIBRARY

Physical Health and Schizophrenia

T0177738

O P L

OXFORD PSYCHIATRY LIBRARY

Physical Health and Schizophrenia

David J. Castle
Professor and Chair of Psychiatry
St Vincent's Hospital
The University of Melbourne
Melbourne, Australia

Peter F. Buckley
Dean
School of Medicine
Virginia Commonwealth University, Richmond, USA

Fiona P. Gaughran
Reader in Psychopharmacology and Physical Health
Institute of Psychiatry, Psychology and Neuroscience
Lead Consultant, National Psychosis Service
Director of R&D
South London and Maudsley NHS Foundation Trust
London, UK

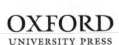

OXFORD
UNIVERSITY PRESS

OXFORD
UNIVERSITY PRESS

Great Clarendon Street, Oxford, OX2 6DP,
United Kingdom

Oxford University Press is a department of the University of Oxford.
It furthers the University's objective of excellence in research, scholarship,
and education by publishing worldwide. Oxford is a registered trade mark of
Oxford University Press in the UK and in certain other countries

Published in the United States of America by Oxford University Press
198 Madison Avenue, New York, NY 10016, United States of America

British Library Cataloguing in Publication Data

Data available

Library of Congress Control Number: 2017943526

ISBN 978–0–19–881168–8

Printed in Great Britain by
Clays Ltd, Elcograf S.p.A.

Oxford University Press makes no representation, express or implied, that the
drug dosages in this book are correct. Readers must therefore always check
the product information and clinical procedures with the most up-to-date
published product information and data sheets provided by the manufacturers
and the most recent codes of conduct and safety regulations. The authors and
the publishers do not accept responsibility or legal liability for any errors in the
text or for the misuse or misapplication of material in this work. Except where
otherwise stated, drug dosages and recommendations are for the non-pregnant
adult who is not breast-feeding

Links to third party websites are provided by Oxford in good faith and
for information only. Oxford disclaims any responsibility for the materials
contained in any third party website referenced in this work.

Foreword

The mind and the body, mental illness, and physical health are intricately intertwined and in bidirectional ways. As mental health professionals, we need to treat the entire person, which includes a focus on functional outcomes, subjective wellbeing, and quality of life. However, to successfully achieve these important goals, we must keep the body in mind. People suffering from schizophrenia also struggle with an earlier onset of physical disorders that reduce their quality of life and functionality and that significantly shorten life expectancy.

In *Physical Health and Schizophrenia*, Castle, Buckley, and Gaughran tackle the complex interaction between schizophrenia and physical health, making a relevant, well-structured, and concise contribution. Through eight chapters, the authors lead the reader from a review of the prevalence of physical comorbidities in people with schizophrenia to the complex contributors to that relationship, including effects of medications, to the mandate of physical health monitoring, and finally to a review of treatment options for the mental health professional and beyond. The book finishes with a very useful Appendix with practical material for mental health professionals, patients, and carers.

The material of this book is made easily digestible by the accessible writing style; relevance of the covered ground that is informed by and addresses key clinical questions; the included rating scales, questionnaires, and monitoring charts, as well as the key point boxes at the beginning of each chapter; and the useful boxes, tables, and figures throughout the book.

I trust that the readers of this book, patients, and carers will each be able to benefit from it.

Christoph U. Correll, MD

Professor of Psychiatry and Molecular Medicine
Hofstra Northwell School of Medicine
Hempstead, NY, USA

Medical Director, Recognition and Prevention (RAP) Program
Department of Psychiatry, The Zucker Hillside Hospital
Northwell Health System
Glen Oaks, NY, USA

Contents

Abbreviations

CDSMP	Chronic Disease Self-Management Program
CI	confidence interval
ECG	electrocardiogram
ECT	electroconvulsive therapy
EPSE	extrapyramidal side effect
GP	general practitioner
HR	hazard ratio
LAI	long-acting injection
LAMIC	low- and middle-income countries
MS	metabolic syndrome
RCT	randomized controlled trial
SMR	standardized mortality ratio
WHO	World Health Organization
WHS	World Health Survey

CHAPTER 1

Physical morbidities and schizophrenia: more than a chance co-occurrence

KEY POINTS

- People with schizophrenia have long carried a major burden of physical health problems.
- There has been a historical tendency to underestimate and undertreat physical health problems among people with schizophrenia.
- Mental health professionals must consider both body and mind to ensure that people with schizophrenia obtain the longevity they deserve.

This book provides an in-depth appraisal of the extent and management of the many physical comorbidities that are seen in people with schizophrenia. The need for such a book as well as the breadth of information contained herein might lead the reader to the conclusion that this association between 'mind' and 'body' in schizophrenia is inextricable and compelling. This has not always appeared so. Rather, the history of serious mental illness is replete with ambiguity and shrouded in public stigma as to whether conditions like schizophrenia are a 'weakness' of the mind or the brain, or both. This chapter sets the scene by providing a brief overview of the schizophrenia concept and its treatments, as well as the association with physical illnesses.

What were early opinions about schizophrenia?

Schizophrenia is a relatively new term, describing a constellation of symptoms and course of illness. Undoubtedly, schizophrenia and other mental illnesses have long existed although in early and medieval times they were ascribed to witchcraft, demonic possession, fevers, plagues, and even an imbalance of humours/bodily fluids. Emil Kraepelin delineated schizophrenia (he termed it 'dementia praecox') from bipolar disorder ('manic depressive insanity') based upon the predominance of certain symptoms and a generally declining course over time. Eugen Bleuler coined the term 'schizophrenia' to describe the fragmentation of mentation and perception that characterize the illness.

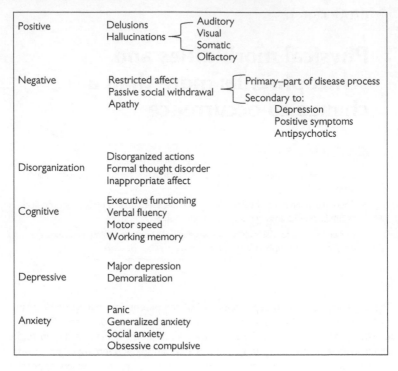

Fig. 1.1 The schizophrenia construct.

Reproduced with permission from Castle D.J. and Buckley P.F., *Schizophrenia*, second edition, figure 2.1, Copyright ©2015 with permission from Oxford University Press.

Our modern conceptualization of the schizophrenia construct recognizes the substantial heterogeneity of both its clinical symptoms and its longitudinal course (Lawrie et al., 2016; Pearlson et al., 2016). A useful conceptual framework for understanding the symptom sets is shown in Fig. 1.1. We will return to this framework when we discuss the overlap between mental and physical problems in people with schizophrenia, and address the contributory causes and barriers to effective care, in Chapter 2.

Why did asylums flourish?

Given the great disability as well as very public manifestations of serious mental illness, the segregation of those afflicted with mental illnesses could be seen as having been both a kindness and a public relief. It was believed that humane treatments, stress-free environments, and fresh air (through walks, meditation in the garden, and farmyard and garden activities) all contributed to a restitution of health of the mind. Quite apparently, it also removed from society individuals whose behaviours were uncontrollable and inherently disturbing. This approach, while ostensibly humane, powerfully fuelled stigma against mental illness and perpetuated the notion that disorders of the mind were different—and should be treated differently and in entirely different healthcare facilities—from physical illnesses.

This approach also ultimately led to a separation of healthcare, with the needs of people with mental illness being met—pretty much exclusively—in large public mental health hospitals. These hospitals—because of the inability to treat adequately, let alone cure, mental illnesses such as schizophrenia—often became a life-long home for people with mental illness (Torrey, 2012). Hence, they became more than just a hospital: they were communities and major industries in their regions. The separation of mental and physical health could not have been more complete.

What was the impact of finding 'real' brain abnormalities in schizophrenia?

Theories of faulty methylation, of serotonergic dysfunction, and dopamine dysregulation all suggested a distinct neurochemical basis for schizophrenia (Nasrallah et al., 2011; Howes et al., 2017). Brain changes in schizophrenia—initially uncovered in post-mortem and early pneumoencephalographic studies—were subtle and inconclusive at best. The advent of computed tomography was astounding for schizophrenia research and confirmed what Kraepelin had suspected all along, namely, that schizophrenia is a brain disorder—the 'dementia of dementia praecox,' as leading British scientists would proclaim in the late 1970s. Perhaps ironically, the confirmation and further discovery of brain abnormalities have also served to sharpen the distinction that schizophrenia is a disorder of the brain and not also of the body.

The aetiopathology of schizophrenia remains enigmatic. Amid theories of dopamine dysregulation and the more modern elaboration of glutamate dysfunction, several other conceptualizations have a more unifying—brain and body—thematic (Howes et al., 2017). There is evidence of abnormal fatty acid metabolism in schizophrenia. There is evidence of inflammation—not just confined to the brain—in schizophrenia. There is genetic evidence of premature ageing in schizophrenia that might confer an overall weakness and predisposition to diseases. There is evidence of mitochondrial dysfunction in schizophrenia and it is intuitive that such an effect would be ubiquitous throughout the body. Even the prevailing theory that schizophrenia is a neurodevelopmental brain disorder also encompasses a faulty development of other issues *in utero* and therefore a more general bodily susceptibility. Thus, while schizophrenia remains enigmatic, the historical divides between mind, brain, and body (that have influenced both research and treatment) appear artificial and even antiquated.

How did treatments for schizophrenia evolve?

A variety of treatments—ranging from outright quackery to thoughtful (yet still misguided) interventions—were used in an attempt to alleviate the suffering of people with schizophrenia. Restraint chairs, bloodletting, bromization, insulin coma, and prefrontal lobotomy, were tried with uncertain outcomes and sometimes further debilitation (Buckley, 2011). Indeed, as late as 1976, it took a seminal study to convince people that kidney dialysis (to remove circulating toxins) was *not* an appropriate treatment for schizophrenia.

In the early part of the last century, with the advent of Freudian psychoanalysis, the treatment of many psychiatric disorders, including schizophrenia, was essentially 'talking therapy'. It was only in the 1930s that the first 'biological' treatment was discovered, namely electroconvulsive therapy (ECT). This was a major breakthrough and undoubtedly helped some patients, but in the days before safe anaesthetic and muscle relaxant regimens it was often traumatic and could be dangerous (of course, modern ECT is a very safe and effective therapy, mostly used for severe depression but also sometimes for treatment-resistant schizophrenia). It was in the early 1950s that the era of modern therapy for schizophrenia was brought in, with the discovery of the calming effects of chlorpromazine. It was this, along with subsequently developed antipsychotic agents, that brought about the closure of asylums and the move towards deinstitutionalization (Buckley, 2011).

So what's all the fuss about the physical health of people with schizophrenia?

Locked away in asylums and with limited access to routine care for physical ailments, the premature death of people with serious mental illnesses was neither disconcerting nor surprising. The often poor physical health environments, overcrowding, and poor sanitation meant infectious diseases were rampant and in the days before antibiotics, often fatal. Nutritional deficiencies led to physical health consequences and could worsen neurocognitive and psychiatric symptoms. And diseases such as syphilis could cause a host of severe and debilitating neuropsychiatric syndromes, giving it the label of 'the great mimic'.

However, with the discovery of antibiotics and major advances in establishing causal organisms for many illness (including syphilis), the overall healthcare of people in asylums should have been expected to improve dramatically. Furthermore, with the advent of antipsychotic medications in the 1950s (see 'How did treatments for schizophrenia evolve?'), many people's mental state improved sufficiently to leave the public mental health facilities, raising the expectation that they could reintegrate into society and live into old age. However, these antipsychotic medications themselves sometimes caused side effects that could contribute to premature death (see Chapter 6). Studies of patterns of physical comorbidities in schizophrenia also led to robust associations with some conditions (e.g. respiratory disorders) and lesser associations with others (e.g. gluten insensitivity) (Miller and Buckley, 2014; Liu et al., 2017).

However, in actuality, the early death of people with schizophrenia continues to the modern day. As outlined elsewhere in this book, numerous studies from around the world have shown that people with schizophrenia die some 15–25 years younger than the general population. This finding was seized upon by advocates and by mental health administrators alike. Additionally, after an initial wave of therapeutic optimism regarding clozapine and other atypical antipsychotic medications, the recognition that these newer agents were somehow contributing to heightened obesity, diabetes, and cardiovascular morbidity was alarming. The realization of a 'physical health crisis' affecting people with schizophrenia was further exacerbated by concerns about perceived commercial gain and potential biases in access to care for the mentally ill. De Hert et al. (2011a) have provided a chastening overview of the extent of physical health problems faced by people living in the twenty-first century with schizophrenia (Box 1.1).

Box 1.1 The extent of physical health problems faced by people with schizophrenia

- Obesity
- Metabolic syndrome
- Diabetes
- Hyperlipidaemia
- Cardiovascular diseases, including hypertension, sudden cardiac death, myocarditis, myocardial infarct, and cerebrovascular disease
- HIV/AIDS
- Hepatic dysfunction, hepatitis B, and hepatitis C
- Tuberculosis, pneumonia, and chronic obstructive pulmonary disease
- Certain cancers
- Osteoporosis and fractures
- Sexual dysfunction, pregnancy and birth complications, and sexually transmitted diseases
- Poor dentition and oral health.

Data from *World Psychiatry*, 10, 2011, De Hert M, Correl CU, Bobes J et al, 'Physical illness in patients with severe mental disorders. I. Prevalence, impact of medications and disparities in health care', pp. 52–77, John Wiley & Sons, Inc.

Box 1.2 Six principles of the WHO *Mental Health Action Plan 2013–2020*

- Universal health coverage
- Human rights
- Evidence-based practice
- Life course approach
- Multisectorial approach
- Empowerment of persons with mental disorders and psychosocial disabilities.

Data from *Mental Health Action Plan 2013–2020*, World Health Organization 2013.

It is encouraging that many health organizations around the world have produced documents and guidelines to assist those in the field to address physical health in people with schizophrenia. For example, the World Health Organization (WHO) has published a useful overarching framework, the *Mental Health Action Plan 2013–2020* (World Health Organization, 2013; Happell et al. 2015) (Box 1.2).

The World Psychiatric Association, through its official journal *World Psychiatry*, has published a number of articles, educational modules, and commentaries that review the relevant literature on physical health problems and early death in people with schizophrenia and provide suggestions as to how clinicians and services can try to address these problems (De Hert et al., 2011a, 2011b; Liu et al., 2017). The field needs to embrace these suggestions and ensure they are delivered on in everyday practice.

Conclusion

This chapter provides a brief historical social overview of schizophrenia as a disorder of both mind and body. Subsequent chapters build on this theme and suggest practical ways in which the continued overabundance of maladies of the body in people with schizophrenia can be appreciated and addressed. As mental health professionals, we must consider both body and mind to ensure our patients obtain the longevity they deserve.

REFERENCES

Buckley PF (2011). Bromization: the truths we know about the psychopharmacology of schizophrenia. *Journal of Nervous and Mental Disease* 199, 736–737.

De Hert M, Correll CU, Bobes J, Cetkovich-Bakmas M, Cohen D, Asai I, et al. (2011a). Physical illness in patients with severe mental disorders. I. Prevalence, impact of medications and disparities in health care. *World Psychiatry* 10, 52–77.

De Hert M, Cohen D, Bobes J, Cetkovich-Bakmas M, Leucht S, Ndetei DM, et al. (2011b). Physical illness in patients with severe mental disorders. II. Barriers to care, monitoring and treatment guidelines, plus recommendations at the system and individual level. *World Psychiatry* 10, 138–151.

Happell B, Platania-Phung C, Webster S, McKenna B, Millar F, Stanton R, et al. (2015). Applying the World Health Organization Mental Health Action Plan to evaluate policy on addressing co-occurrence of physical and mental illness in Australia. *Australian Health Review* 39, 370–378.

Howes OD, McCutcheon R, Own MJ, Murray RM (2017). The role of genes, stress, and dopamine in the development of schizophrenia. *Biological Psychiatry* 81, 9–20.

Lawrie SM, O'Donovan MC, Saks E, Burns T, Lieberman JA (2016). Improving classification of psychoses. *Lancet Psychiatry* 3, 367–374.

Liu NH, Daumit GL, Dua T, Aquila R, Charlson F, Cuijpers P, et al. (2017). Excess mortality in persons with severe mental disorders: a multilevel intervention framework and priorities for clinical guidance, policy and research agendas. *World Psychiatry* 16, 30–40.

Miller B, Buckley PF (2014). Medical and psychiatric comorbidities: complicating treatment expectations. In: Buckley PF, Gaughran F (eds) *Treatment-Refractory Schizophrenia: A Clinical Conundrum*, pp. 45–63. Berlin: Springer.

Nasrallah H, Tandon R, Keshavan M (2011). Beyond the facts in schizophrenia: closing the gaps in diagnosis, pathophysiology, and treatment. *Epidemiology and Psychiatric Sciences* 20, 317–327.

Pearlson GD, Clementz BA, Sweeney JA, Keshavan MS, Tamminga CA (2016). Does biology transcend the symptom-based boundaries of psychosis? *Psychiatric Clinics of North America* 39, 165–174.

Torrey EF (2012). *The Insanity Offense: How America's Failure to Treat the Seriously Mentally Ill Endangers Its Citizens*. New York: WW Norton & Company.

World Health Organization (2013). *Mental Health Action Plan 2013–2020*. Geneva: World Health Organization.

REFERENCES

CHAPTER 2

Reasons for excess medical morbidity in schizophrenia

> **KEY POINTS**
>
> - People with schizophrenia are at high risk of a number of different physical health problems. Reasons for this excess risk are complex, and encompass individual and service-related factors.
> - Clinicians should be aware of these excess risks and the drivers thereof, and endeavour to address them holistically.

Chapter 1 has outlined the extent of excess physical health morbidity and early mortality in people with schizophrenia. In this chapter, we try to understand the factors contributing to this serious state of affairs. We consider the following in turn: shared aetiological factors, illness-related factors, personal issues, and system issues. Factors related to the use of psychotropic medications and their contribution to the risk of metabolic syndrome in particular are touched on only briefly as this topic is covered in detail in Chapters 3 and 6.

Shared aetiological factors

It is intriguing that historical reports of elevated rates of physical health problems in people with schizophrenia—notably elements of the metabolic syndrome—antedate the introduction of antipsychotic medications. Also, in some but not all studies, some of these factors appear to afflict individuals even before the onset of frank psychosis—and certainly before the prescription of antipsychotics. For example, Cohen and De Hert (2011), in a population-based study in Denmark, reported that individuals just diagnosed with schizophrenia and before treatment had been instituted, had an elevated risk of diabetes of 1.27–1.63 times the general population at the same age (mean 29 years). Furthermore, Ryan et al. (2003) showed unmedicated first-episode patients to have higher levels of plasma glucose, as well as impaired glucose tolerance and more insulin resistance, than general population controls. A recent meta-analysis of 911 antipsychotic-naïve patients and 870 controls largely confirmed the finding of heightened insulin resistance and impaired glucose tolerance (Greenhalgh et al., 2017).

This evidence of an underlying vulnerability among people with early psychosis—and before exposure to antipsychotics—to perturbations in

> **Box 2.1** Shared aetiological mechanisms in schizophrenia and cardiovascular disease
>
> ● Common *genetic factors* (e.g. between schizophrenia and type 2 diabetes).
> ● *Neurotransmitters* involved in the pathogenesis of schizophrenia (e.g. dopamine, serotonin, and histamine) also have peripheral effects on the pancreas and adipocytes.
> ● *Stress hormones* (notably cortisol) are elevated in early psychosis and are implicated in cardiovascular risk.
> ● *Immune mechanisms and inflammatory pathways* appear to play a role in schizophrenia as well as cardiovascular risk.
>
> Data from *Frontiers in Psychiatry*, 5, 2014, Ringen PA, Engh JA, Birkenaes AB et al, 'Increased mortality in schizophrenia due to cardiovascular disease—a non-systematic review of epidemiology, possible causes, and interventions', Frontiers Media.

metabolic homeostasis, begs the question as to whether there are shared risk factors for both metabolic abnormalities and schizophrenia. Converging lines of research suggest that this is indeed likely. These factors have recently been reviewed by Ringen et al. (2014) and are summarized in Box 2.1. An important caveat is that this does not necessarily mean that the lack of a family history of a physical disease reduces the likelihood of an adverse cardiovascular risk outcome upon exposure to antipsychotics: indeed, Foley et al. (2015) reported that an increased risk of diabetes associated with a range of antipsychotic agents was seen only in individuals *without* a family risk of diabetes.

Illness-related factors

The symptoms of schizophrenia are neatly conceptualized as shown in Box 2.2. Each set of symptoms impact the individual in terms of healthy living and can be a barrier to effective healthcare.

Positive symptoms such as persecutory beliefs can lead to avoidance of crowds and noise, reducing the likelihood of regular outdoor activities and gym attendance.

Disorganization symptoms can render the individual compromised in terms of their ability to organize daily activities such as attending medical appointments, performing regular exercise, or cooking healthy food.

Negative symptoms include apathetic social withdrawal and a lack of drive, which directly impact engagement in physical activities. Negative symptoms also seem to drive nicotine and other substance misuse.

Cognitive dysfunction is common in people with schizophrenia and affects a number of domains, as shown in Box 2.2. These cognitive problems can impede engagement in work and studies, adding to social isolation and low income, which in turn are associated with poor diet and lifestyle.

Box 2.2 Domains of cognitive functioning impaired in schizophrenia

Mild impairment
- Perception skills
- Delayed recognition memory
- Verbal and full-scale IQ.

Moderate impairment
- Distractibility
- Memory and working memory
- Delayed recall.

Severe impairment
- Executive functioning
- Verbal fluency
- Motor speed.

Reproduced from Wykes T and Castle D, 'Cognition'. In DJ Castle, D Copolov, T Wykes, K Mueser, eds. *Pharmacological and Psychosocial Treatments for Schizophrenia*, 3rd ed. Copyright (2007) with permission from Taylor & Francis Group, Informa UK Limited.

Depression is also common in people with schizophrenia and can be associated with apathy and withdrawal and a lack of motivation, reducing the likelihood of regular exercise. In some forms of depression there is carbohydrate craving and weight gain.

Anxiety, notably *social anxiety*, can also impede socialization and deter people from engagement in group activities. Some people with *panic disorder* avoid exercise for fear of precipitating a panic attack.

Personal issues

People with schizophrenia are generally not well placed to engage in healthy lifestyles, in part due to illness factors (see 'Illness-related factors'); in part as a consequence of poor financial means; and in part due to lack of availability of appropriate opportunities.

There is, for example, a high rate of *sedentary behaviours* among people with schizophrenia, driven in part by negative symptoms but also by apathy and fatigue (possibly compounded by sedative antipsychotics) and by depression. Anxiety, personal stigma, embarrassment about obesity, and cost might be barriers to regular attendance at gyms or public swimming pools. And the stark fact is that many people with schizophrenia simply don't have any reason to get out of their home. They all too often have restricted social networks and little peer or family support.

A *healthy diet* is increasingly seen as a key component of good physical health. There is good evidence that a Mediterranean-style diet (see Box A.1 in the

Appendix) is particularly useful for good cardiovascular health. There is emerging evidence that it can help ameliorate depressed mood as well (Jacka et al., 2017), albeit we are aware of no studies specifically in depressed people with schizophrenia. The problem with this diet, however, is that it is fairly expensive, with oily fish such as salmon and olive oil being out of reach of many people with schizophrenia.

People with schizophrenia tend to have high-caloric diets with relatively poor nutritional value (Simonelli-Muñoz et al., 2012). 'Carbohydrate craving' can be a consequence of some antipsychotic medications (see Chapter 6) and can also be seen in association with negative symptoms and depressed mood. Hahn et al. (2014), in a sample of 1286 adults with psychosis, found that 74% ate fewer than four servings of fruit and vegetables daily: this was associated with less frequent meals and higher use of high- versus low-fat milk, adding salt to food, lower levels of physical activity, and more sedentary behaviour. Thus, there were a number of inter-related factors adding to the cardiovascular risk burden. In multiple regression modelling, current use of tobacco, and alcohol and cannabis abuse were associated with lower fruit and vegetable intake, underlining the complex interaction of risk factors.

The use of *tobacco, alcohol,* and *illicit substances* is common among people with schizophrenia. The reasons are complex and multifaceted, encompassing social, behavioural, cognitive, and biological reward domains. Suffice to say here that these behaviours carry myriad physical health risks in and of themselves (e.g. smoking with chronic obstructive pulmonary disease, lung and other cancers; alcohol with hepatic cirrhosis and its attendant complications as well as peripheral neuropathy, central nervous system damage, cardiomyopathy, and numerous other physical health problems) but are also associated with indirect effects on physical health problems. For example, alcohol abuse is often associated with nutritional insufficiencies and unsafe injecting of illicit drugs can cause local infections at injection sites, endocarditis, hepatitis C, and HIV/AIDS. Behaviours associated with substance misuse include risky sexual behaviours that leave individuals at risk of a range of sexually transmitted diseases, some of which can leave women infertile or, in the case of HIV/AIDS, can result in expensive lifelong complex treatment regimens or even prove fatal.

System issues

As outlined in Chapters 1 and 8 of this book, there are fundamental system issues that bedevil comprehensive physical and mental healthcare provision for people with schizophrenia. Of course, jurisdictions differ in regard to how they set up services to help people with chronic mental illnesses, and no doubt some do it better than others, but it is fair to say that in many countries there are significant gaps: indeed, in some countries there are practically no dedicated resources for the mentally ill or policies to guide care (de Hert et al., 2011).

Health systems are almost always fragmented and complex to negotiate. There are added issues for people with schizophrenia to understand and navigate these complex systems, as outlined earlier. There are also financial barriers to accessing healthcare providers as well as to treatments.

Added to these issues is that physical health systems are often simply not set up well to offer the best care to people with schizophrenia and related disorders, even if they do manage to get access to the appropriate part of the system. The literature is replete with examples of how people with such illnesses are disadvantaged in this regard. In a recent review, Moore et al. (2015) provide a number of such instances, as shown in Box 2.3 (see Moore et al. (2015) for further information).

Not all the examples provided in Box 2.3 are directly caused by deficits in physical healthcare provision, but they should serve as a reminder of the biases and barriers that do exist. The general issue of relatively poor provision of physical healthcare for people with schizophrenia is reflected in an important record linkage study in Western Australia, where Lawrence et al. (2013) confirmed high relative rates of a number of physical health problems among people with illnesses such as schizophrenia, but starkly highlight that it is not merely the increased rate of disease but the even higher increase in rate of death from such diseases that point to deficits in physical health service provision for this vulnerable group. At a broader level, it is chastening that, whilst greater longevity is being achieved for the general population in most countries of the world, the earlier death among people with schizophrenia is relatively static, resulting in a widening gap.

Box 2.3 Examples of health provision inequalities for people with schizophrenia

- Low rates of screening for cardiovascular risk factors.
- Lower rates of screening for osteoporosis, blood pressure and cholesterol monitoring, vaccinations, and mammography.
- For people with schizophrenia who develop diabetes, lower rates of routine eye checks and poorer glycaemic control.
- Lower rates of prescription of cardiovascular drugs, notably lipid-lowering and antihypertensive agents.
- Worse outcomes for people with a wide range of cancers, with lower rates of surgical interventions and radiotherapy, and fewer sessions of chemotherapy.
- Higher mortality rates following major bone fractures and higher odds of postoperative complications following hip or knee arthroplasty.
- Very high rates of poor dentition, with edentulous status being much higher than in the general population.

Conclusion

There are numerous reasons why people with schizophrenia are at high risk of a number of different physical health problems and are more likely to die young, compared with the general population.

REFERENCES

Cohen D, De Hert M (2011). Endogenic and iatrogenic diabetes mellitus in drug-naïve schizophrenia: the role of olanzapine and its place in the psychopharmacology treatment algorithm. *Neuropsychopharmacology* 36, 2368–2369.

De Hert M, Cohen D, Bobes J, Cetkovich-Bakmas M, Leucht S, Ndetei DM, et al. (2011). Physical illness in patients with severe mental disorders. II. Barriers to care, monitoring and treatment guidelines, plus recommendations at the system and individual level. *World Psychiatry* 10, 138–151.

Foley D, Mackinnon A, Morgan V, Watts GF, Castle DJ, Waterreus A, Galletly C (2015). Effect of age, family history of diabetes, and antipsychotic drug treatment on risk of diabetes in people with psychosis: a population-based cross-sectional study. *Lancet Psychiatry* 2, 1092–1098.

Greenhalgh AM, Gonzalez-Blanco L, Garcia-Rizo C, Fernandez-Egea E, Miller B, Arroyo MB, Kirkpatrick B (2017). Meta-analysis of glucose intolerance, insulin, and insulin resistance in antipsychotic-naïve patients with nonaffective psychosis. *Schizophrenia Research* 179, 57–63.

Hahn LA, Galletly CA, Foley DL, Mackinnon A, Watts GF, Castle DJ, et al. (2014). Inadequate fruit and vegetable intake in people with psychosis. *Australia and New Zealand Journal of Psychiatry* 48, 1025–1035.

Jacka FN, O'Neil A, Opie R, Itsiopoulos C, Cotton S, Mohebbi M, et al. (2017). A randomised controlled trial of dietary improvement for adults with major depression (the 'SMILES' trial). *BMC Medicine* 15, 23.

Lawrence DM, Hancock KJ, Kisely S (2013). The gap in life expectancy from preventable physical illness in Western Australia: retrospective analysis of population-based registers. *BMJ* 346, f2539.

Moore S, Shiers D, Daly B, Mitchell AJ, Gaughran F (2015). Promoting physical health for people with schizophrenia by reducing disparities in medical and dental care. *Acta Psychiatrica Scandinavica* 132, 109–121.

Ringen PA, Engh JA, Birkenaes AB, Dieset I, Andreassen OA (2014). Increased mortality in schizophrenia due to cardiovascular disease—a non-systematic review of epidemiology, possible causes, and interventions. *Frontiers in Psychiatry* 5, 137.

Ryan MC, Collins P, Thakore JH (2003). Impaired fasting glucose tolerance in first-episode, drug-naïve patients with schizophrenia. *American Journal of Psychiatry* 160, 284–289.

Simonelli-Muñoz AJ, Fortea MI, Solario P, Gallego-Gomez JI, Sánchez-Bautista S, Balanza S (2012). Dietary habits of patients with schizophrenia: a self-reported questionnaire survey. *International Journal of Mental Health Nursing* 21, 220–228.

CHAPTER 3

The metabolic syndrome in schizophrenia

KEY POINTS

- The metabolic syndrome (MS) is seen in excess among people with schizophrenia.
- The reasons are complex but encompass underlying (genetic) predisposition as well as lifestyle factors.
- Antipsychotic medications can also add to the risk, and some tend to do so to a greater degree than others.
- The risk of MS must be borne in mind when treating people with schizophrenia and particularly in terms of choice of antipsychotic agent.
- People with schizophrenia deserve the very best treatments for their physical health.

The metabolic syndrome (MS) is a constellation of obesity and related metabolic abnormalities that predict poor cardiovascular and overall health status. While various diagnostic criteria for MS have been proposed and validated in general (non-psychiatric) populations, common to all of these are the five criteria shown in Box 3.1. Three of the five criteria are required for the diagnosis of MS. The health consequences of MS and associated heightened risks for other physical comorbidities include diabetes, cardiovascular and heart disease, retinal disease, liver disease, pulmonary diseases (especially sleep apnoea), and osteoarthritis (Aguilar et al., 2015; Vancampfort et al., 2015).

How common is MS?

There is concern, worldwide, that the incidence of MS and its associated health conditions—obesity, diabetes—is increasing. The rate of MS among the US young adult population aged 20–29 years old is 6.7% (Aguilar et al., 2015). There has been a disproportionate rise in the rates of MS among patients with schizophrenia, an occurrence that has aggravated already substantial physical comorbidities in psychosis (Miller and Buckley, 2014; Henderson et al., 2015). In the landmark US Clinical Antipsychotic Trials of Intervention Effectiveness (CATIE) study of approximately 1200 adult patients with chronic schizophrenia, 40% of patients met the criteria for MS. In a comparable study (Comparison of Atypicals for First

> **Box 3.1** Criteria for metabolic syndrome
>
> - Increased waist circumference
> - High blood pressure
> - Elevating fasting blood glucose
> - Elevated triglycerides
> - Low high-density lipoprotein cholesterol level.

Episode (CAFE)) of 400 patients with first-episode schizophrenia, 4.3% met the criteria for MS at baseline and treatment-emergent MS, was listed in 13.4% of patients over the 1-year treatment trial (Patel et al., 2009). In another US study of first-episode schizophrenia—the Recovery After an Initial Schizophrenia Episode (RAISE)—MS was recorded among 13.2% of patients (Correll et al., 2014). Moreover, prediabetes (based upon fasting elevated glucose levels) and diabetes were noted in 4% and 3% of patients, respectively.

In a British study (Improving Physical Health and Reducing Substance Use in Severe Mental Illness (IMPaCT)) of 450 adults with schizophrenia, the rate of MS was 56.8% (Gardner-Sood et al., 2015). Interestingly, 8 of 13 patients who had not received antipsychotic medications also met the criteria for MS. In the European 1-year first-episode study (EUFEST), 6% of 498 patients met MS criteria at entry to the study and 58% had at least one pre-existing MS risk factor (Fleischhacker et al., 2013). In an Australian study, a MS rate of 57% was observed among schizophrenia patients receiving clozapine (Galletly et al., 2012). All in all, the majority of studies find rates of MS in patients with schizophrenia are in excess of those of the general population and that this risk is present even early in the course of illness.

What causes MS?

In the general population, MS is associated with both genetic and environmental (lifestyle, nutritional, activity) risk factors. There is also a complex and intriguing scientific story that relates MS to inflammation (Henderson et al., 2015; Mori et al., 2016). In an analysis from the CATIE study, blood C-reactive protein (CRP), interleukin-6, leptin, total white cell count, and total lymphocyte count predicted the presence of MS (Mori et al., 2016).

The extent to which various causative factors apply to people with schizophrenia who develop MS is a keen focus of current research, particularly in view of the raised rates of MS among patients who receive second-generation antipsychotic medications. For example, several studies point to a higher rate of diabetes in the relatives of patients with schizophrenia, and these suggest a shared familial risk rather than a diabetogenic effect of antipsychotic medications. The reader is referred to Chapter 2 of this book for a more detailed discussion of these factors.

MS and antipsychotic medication: what is the relationship?

An early study following up on patients who had received 10 years of treatment with clozapine showed 43% had new-onset diabetes (Henderson et al., 2015). This was a staggering finding. Then, with other studies reporting new-onset diabetes during treatment with newer antipsychotic medications, along with studies showing rapid and substantial weight gain on some such agents, concerns were raised that the advent and use of second-generation antipsychotics had, of themselves, caused a rush of new-onset MS. The passage of time as well as more carefully conducted treatment studies started to point to a more complex relationship. This includes 'host–drug' interactions, namely the same risk factors for MS that are evident in the non-psychiatric, general population, and then the relative propensity of each antipsychotic to induce MS (Vancampfort et al., 2015).

Biological studies trying to determine the cause of the weight gain and other metabolic side effects of the atypical agents have enriched our understanding of the causation of MS broadly and it is clear that individual factors also play a role in that some people simply do not gain weight, for example, on medications that in clinical trials tend to be associated with substantial weight gain. We are not yet able to predict who will and who will not be at heightened risk of MS in association with which drugs, but a general 'rank order' of the propensity to MS is shown in Table 3.1. These issues are discussed further in Chapter 6.

Table 3.1 Risk of metabolic syndrome and weight gain associated with antipsychotic medications[a]

Higher risk	Clozapine
	Olanzapine
	Quetiapine
Moderate risk	Risperidone
	Paliperidone
Lower risk	Ziprasidone
	Aripiprazole
	Lurasidone
	Asenapine

[a] This schema represents the authors' interpretation of risk and relative risk across currently available antipsychotics; others might order these differently.

What can be done to prevent MS?

Just as in the general adult population, early identification and preventative measures are key in avoiding or ameliorating the risk of MS (Gardner-Sood et al., 2015; Moore et al., 2015). This is perhaps even more so for people with schizophrenia since, while not consistent across all available studies, the present information on MS rates among high-risk, prodromal populations show comparable MS rates to the general population. This suggests that preventive strategies might indeed be feasible.

For first-episode patients and patients with chronic schizophrenia, the prevention of MS involves lifestyle changes as well as judicious decisions about the selection and use of antipsychotic medications. These issues are now 'front and centre' in the psychopharmacology and care of people with schizophrenia and are covered in detail in Chapters 6 and 8 of this book.

What are the behaviour and lifestyle management strategies to address MS in schizophrenia?

In general, approaches to the management of MS in people with schizophrenia mirror those of MS care in the general population (Box 3.2). Moreover—and perhaps surprisingly given the many mitigating factors—implementing lifestyle and behavioural changes to reduce weight, improve nutrition, and increase exercise can achieve broadly comparable outcomes in people with schizophrenia to those in the general population. That said, losing weight and changing one's diet is challenging for the best of patients with MS and so the actual results of weight

---

Box 3.2 Comprehensive physical healthcare for people with schizophrenia

- Nutritional support and education
- Preventative screenings and immunizations
- Access to family medicine-internal medicine services
- Integrated (co-located) healthcare for physical and mental health needs
- Health coaches and peer support
- Safe and supportive housing
- Disability and healthcare insurances—parity between medical and mental health components
- Medication insurance and financial aid
- Psychiatric drugs
- Other medicines
- Dental health
- Sexual education, counselling, and sexual healthcare
- Integrated psychogeriatric care
- Tailored palliative care.

reduction studies in schizophrenia through lifestyle changes show only modest results. Several studies have tailored nutritional and exercise programmes—already of proven benefit in large-scale cardiovascular and obesity management studies in the general population—to patients with schizophrenia where instructional details and duration of interventions are less complex (Moore et al., 2015). For further details, the reader is referred to Chapter 8.

Another very important healthcare approach is to reduce the disparities in healthcare for people with schizophrenia and to increase their access to high-quality medical care in tandem with their mental healthcare. There are many approaches to this, including enhanced access to medical clinics and, alternatively, co-locating medical clinics in/with/beside psychiatric outpatient clinics. Integrated healthcare is now an evolving strategy for managing the physical comorbidities—including MS—in patients with schizophrenia (Miller and Buckley, 2014). These approaches are covered in detail in Chapter 8, while patient information material is provided in the Appendix.

What is the value of medications in treating MS in schizophrenia?

In general, people with schizophrenia who develop MS and do not reduce their risk despite exercise and dietary interventions deserve the option of treatment with lipid-lowering and other agents as would be used in people without schizophrenia. Regrettably, the rate of prescription of such agents is lower in people with schizophrenia than those without: another indication of the gap in healthcare provision for this vulnerable group. For example, in the Australian Study of High Impact Psychosis (Galletly et al., 2012), the majority of people with risk factors for MS (elevated fasting glucose and lipids; hypertension) were not receiving treatment for these and those who were, were mostly suboptimally treated.

Specific strategies to help deal with particular components of MS are detailed in Chapters 6 and 8. Suffice to say here that the early use of metformin is proving popular as a safe and easy way to help reduce or prevent at least some weight gain (albeit only a few kilograms) and reduce insulin sensitivity. Statins can generally be used without particular problems in people on antipsychotics, but, as with all medications, drug–drug interactions need to be explored before prescribing. Some evidence also supports the use of topiramate for weight loss as well as melatonin. Antihypertensive medication prescription should generally follow the guidelines provided for the general population, with extra care regarding drug–drug interactions and potential psychiatric side effects of some antihypertensives (e.g. depression with beta-blockers).

Clinical opinion is divided as to when to introduce these drugs, with some prescribers even suggesting that metformin and statins should be given proactively when patients commence antipsychotic therapy as 'prophylaxis'. Beyond complexity of care and exposure to potential adverse effects of some of these agents, the cost of these drugs for an already financially overburdened mental healthcare system should also be taken into consideration, albeit there is no excuse for systematic bias against prescribing effective agents to people with schizophrenia.

Conclusion

MS is seen in excess among people with schizophrenia. The reasons are complex but encompass underlying (genetic) predisposition as well as lifestyle factors. Antipsychotic medications can also add to the risk, and some tend to do so to a greater degree than others. Risk of MS must be borne in mind when treating people with schizophrenia and particularly in terms of choice of antipsychotic agent. People with schizophrenia deserve the very best treatments for their physical health and should not be denied effective treatment options available for components of MS, merely because they have schizophrenia.

REFERENCES

Aguilar M, Bhuket T, Torres S, Liu B, Wong RJ (2015). Prevalence of the metabolic syndrome in the United States, 2003–2012. *JAMA* 313(19), 1973–1974.

Correll CU, Robinson DG, Schooler NR, Brunette MF, Mueser KT, Rosenhek RA, et al. (2014). Cardiometabolic risk in patients with first episode schizophrenia spectrum disorders: baseline results from the RAISE-ETP study. *JAMA Psychiatry* 7(12), 1350–1363.

Fleischhacker WW, Siu CO, Boden R, Pappadopuulos E, Karayal ON, Kahn RS; EUFEST study group (2013). Metabolic risk factors in first episode schizophrenia: baseline prevalence and course analyzed from the European First- Episode Schizophrenia Trial. *International Journal of Neuropsychopharmacology* 16(5), 987–995.

Galletly C, Foley D, Waterreus A, Watts G, Castle D, McGrath J, et al. (2012). Cardiometabolic risk factors in people with psychosis: the second Australian national survey of psychosis. *Australian & New Zealand Journal of Psychiatry* 46, 753–761.

Gardner-Sood P, Lally J, Smith S, Atakan Z, Ismail K, Greenwood KE, et al. (2015). Cardiovascular risk factors and metabolic syndrome in people with established psychotic illnesses: baseline data from the IMPaCT randomized controlled trial. *Psychological Medicine* 48, 2619–2629.

Henderson DC, Vincenzi B, Andrea NV, Ulloa M, Copeland PM (2015). Pathophysiological mechanisms of increased cardiometabolic risk in people with schizophrenia and other severe mental illnesses. *Lancet Psychiatry* 2(5), 452–464.

Miller B, Buckley PF (2014). Medical and psychiatric comorbidities: complicating treatment expectations. In: Buckley PF, Gaughran F (eds) *Treatment-Refractory Schizophrenia: A Clinical Conundrum*, pp. 45–63. Berlin: Springer.

Moore S, Shiers D, Daly B, Mitchell AJ, Gaughran F (2015). Promoting physical health for people with schizophrenia by reducing disparities in medical and dental care. *Acta Psychiatrica Scandinavica* 132, 109–121.

Mori N, McEvoy JP, Miller BJ (2016). Total and differential white blood cell counts, inflammatory markers, adipokines, and the metabolic syndrome in phase 1 of the clinical antipsychotic trials of intervention effectiveness study. *Schizophrenia Research* 169, 30–35.

Patel JK, Buckley PF, Hamer RM, Woolson S, McEvoy JP, Perkins D, Lieberman JA (2009). Metabolic profiles of second-generation antipsychotics in early psychosis: findings from the CAFE study. *Schizophrenia Research* 111(1–3), 9–16.

Vancampfort D, Stubbs B, Mitchell AJ, De Hert M, Wampers M, Ward PB, et al. (2015). Risk of metabolic syndrome and its components in people with schizophrenia and related psychotic disorders, bipolar disorder and major depressive disorder; a systematic review and meta-analysis. *World Psychiatry* 14, 339–347.

CHAPTER 4

Other physical health problems in people with schizophrenia

KEY POINTS

- People with schizophrenia are at high risk of developing many physical health conditions.
- Outcomes for physical health problems are generally worse for people with schizophrenia than the general population.
- The disorganization dimension of psychosis and cognitive problems may mean that setting up appointments with healthcare professionals may be a challenge without support.
- Disorganization and cognitive and motivational difficulties may make complex treatment regimens difficult to put into practice.
- Healthcare professionals should make reasonable adjustments to provide equity in the physical healthcare of people with psychotic illnesses.

Much of the work on premature mortality in schizophrenia has focused on cardiovascular disease (Chapter 3) and modifiable risk factors, including tobacco smoking (Chapter 5). However, cardiovascular disease is not the only cause of early death in schizophrenia. Olfson et al. (2015) examined mortality in the US Medicaid programme, the largest funder of health services for people with schizophrenia across the US. Natural causes accounted for most of the deaths, of which cardiovascular disease made up one-third. Approximately one-sixth of natural deaths were as a result of cancer, with lung cancer having the highest mortality rate, especially in older men of white ethnicity. Overall, people with schizophrenia had a much higher standardized mortality ratio (SMR) than did controls (all-cause SMR, 3.7; 95% confidence interval (CI), 3.7–3.7). The SMR was higher for women than men, and for older adults and those of white ethnicity compared to other ethnic groups. There were markedly raised SMRs for cardiovascular disease (3.6; 95% CI, 3.5–3.6), diabetes (4.2; 95% CI, 4.0–4.3) (especially in younger adults), chronic obstructive pulmonary disease (9.9; 95% CI, 9.6–10.2), and influenza/pneumonia (7.0; 95% CI, 6.7–7.4). Moore et al. (2015) have summarized some of the reasons for such morbidity among people with psychotic disorders, as summarized in Table 4.1.

Table 4.1 Reasons for excess mortality and wider morbidity in psychosis	
Wider determinants of health	Urban living Poverty Unemployment
Individual biological factors	Shared genetic risk for cardiovascular disease or diabetes Shared risk for autoimmunity
Factors related to illness	Active psychosis impairs ability to communicate symptoms succinctly Cognitive dysfunction impairs ability to follow complex treatment plan
Lifestyle factors	Smoking Sedentary behaviour Poor diet
Antipsychotic medication	Acute effects on electrocardiogram (QTc interval) Longer-term effects on weight gain, glucose and lipid metabolism, and bone health
Quality of care	
Prevention	Reduced uptake of screening, e.g. mammography, blood pressure
Long-term condition management	Incomplete screening and intervention for cardiometabolic risk in psychosis Inequitable application of best evidence in pharmacological management
Acute care	Less interventional treatments after acute cardiac events

Data from *Acta Psychiatrica Scandinavica*, 11, 2015, Moore S, Daly B, Shiers D et al, 'Promoting physical health by reducing disparities in medical and dental care'.

This chapter provides a brief overview of physical health maladies associated with schizophrenia, other than metabolic syndrome, which is covered in Chapter 3. We do not deal specifically with problems associated with antipsychotic medications, as that topic is addressed in Chapter 6.

One physical health problem at a time?

Regrettably, it appears that many physical health problems occur together in people with schizophrenia, resulting in added complexity and disease and treatment burden at an individual level. Thus, a recent study of 242,952 people from 48 low- and middle-income countries (LMIC) recruited through the World Health

Survey (WHS) examined nine physical disorders, namely arthritis, angina pectoris, asthma, diabetes, chronic back pain, visual impairment, hearing problems, edentulism, and tuberculosis. Multimorbidity (i.e. two or more physical health comorbidities) was seen in 11% of controls but in 36% of those with psychotic disorders. Multimorbidity is associated with functional decline and poorer quality of life as well as with early death (Stubbs et al., 2016a).

The WHS study also underlines the particular burden of physical health problems in LMIC, where there is a dearth of medical facilities, often poor living conditions, and high rates of social disadvantage. Indeed, in some such jurisdictions old-style large asylums still operate, with concomitant poor nutrition, overcrowding, and vulnerability to infectious diseases such as tuberculosis (Sharan, 2017).

What is the burden of pulmonary problems in people with schizophrenia?

Chronic obstructive pulmonary disease, pneumonia, and influenza are major causes of disability and death in people with schizophrenia. This is not entirely unexpected, given the array of risk factors such as smoking, obesity, and sedentary behaviour. Furthermore, antipsychotics have been linked to acute respiratory failure in people with chronic obstructive pulmonary disease, so it is possible that they may have a similar compromising effect on lung heath in people taking them for their primary indication, psychosis (Wang et al., 2017). Clozapine, the antipsychotic used in resistant psychosis, has a particular association with pneumonia in some people.

Even though the SMRs for both influenza and cardiac events are elevated in people with schizophrenia, influenza vaccination is not offered routinely to them. There is also a problem, worse in LMIC, of other infectious pulmonary diseases, notably tuberculosis. The high rates of HIV/AIDS in some such jurisdictions make people expressly vulnerable to such infectious diseases. Further work is needed to develop evidence-based clinical systems to assess and promote lung health in people with schizophrenia.

Bones, falls, and fractures

Bone health is a major problem for people with schizophrenia, as evidenced by the high rate of fractures, with an incidence rate ratio of 1.72 compared to controls (Stubbs et al., 2015b). There are many risk factors for falls, such as antipsychotic medication, distraction, pain, and poor coordination; and when a fall occurs, bone strength is compromised. There are number of different reasons for this.

Firstly, many antipsychotics increase serum levels of prolactin, which is likely to confer a longer-term risk of osteoporosis (see Chapter 6). This risk is compounded by the high rates of overweight and obesity, tobacco smoking, and sedentary behaviour. Certainly, bone mineral density is lower in both the hip and lumbar spine regions in people with schizophrenia compared to healthy controls (Gomez et al., 2016).

Vitamin D is important for bone health. Vitamin D is mainly acquired from exposure of the skin to sunlight with a small proportion absorbed through diet. Given the lack of socialization and outdoor activities, as well as poor nutrition, it is hardly surprising that people with schizophrenia often have low vitamin D levels. Almost half of people with established psychosis are vitamin D deficient, while people experiencing their first episode of psychosis are three times more likely to be vitamin D deficient than controls matched for age, sex, and ethnicity (Crews et al., 2013). We do not know whether these patients had a pre-morbid vitamin D deficiency, which would influence bone health as well as affecting the chance of developing schizophrenia in the first place, in that people who have low vitamin D levels at birth are more likely to develop schizophrenia in adult life (McGrath et al., 2010).

Overall, hyperprolactinaemia, low vitamin D levels, prolonged periods of sedentary behaviour, prolonged hospitalizations, tobacco smoking, and obesity together result in a reduction in bone integrity and a higher risk of fracture. These are summarized in Fig. 4.1. Advice about bone health, including exercise and nutritional programmes, is required, as is the

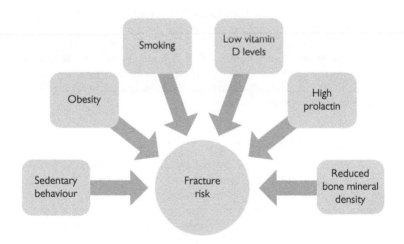

Fig. 4.1 Bone health vulnerabilities in schizophrenia.

monitoring of prolactin levels in people prescribed antipsychotics (see Chapter 6).

Autoimmunity and schizophrenia

The relationship between schizophrenia and autoimmunity has been examined over the decades (Benros et al., 2014), but is of particular interest in recent years, especially since we became aware that disease-relevant autoantibodies, such as those against N-methyl-D-aspartic acid or voltage-gated potassium channels, may induce psychotic symptoms. At a more general level, having schizophrenia increases the chance of developing an autoimmune disease by about half while reciprocally, a personal or family history of autoimmune disease increases the chance of developing schizophrenia.

Particular epidemiological associations have been reported between schizophrenia and coeliac disease, Graves' disease, psoriasis, pernicious anaemia, and autoimmune hepatitis. Intriguingly, there appears to be an additional environmental effect, such that if someone with an autoimmune disease also has a hospital admission for infection, then their risk of psychosis is further magnified (Benros et al., 2014).

There have been a number of reports of a negative association between schizophrenia and rheumatoid arthritis. This is interesting, as a Danish population study found that this negative association was not limited to rheumatoid arthritis alone but was evident with other degenerative musculoskeletal conditions (Mors et al., 1999). It is therefore possible that the sedentary lifestyle so common in people with psychosis means that rheumatoid arthritis, along with other conditions that affect movement, is simply not brought to the attention of doctors.

Do we ask about snoring?

People with schizophrenia often report poor sleep or altered sleep patterns, such as daytime somnolence. Often this is seen as a symptom of schizophrenia. However, if a history of snoring is elicited, especially if the person is overweight or has other risk factors, then consideration should be given to a diagnosis of obstructive sleep apnoea.

People with schizophrenia have higher rates of obstructive sleep apnoea than controls (Stubbs et al., 2016b). As outlined in Chapter 6, sedative antipsychotics and other medications can contribute to diurnal sedation, and weight gain can exacerbate obstructive sleep apnoea. Specific questioning about sleep quality, nocturnal awakenings, and snoring (along with corroboration from a sleeping partner, if possible), can help make the diagnosis, which can be confirmed with polysomnography. Involvement of a sleep physician and institution of therapeutic measures such as dental appliances (though poor dentition can be a problem with these) or continuous positive airway pressure machines should be considered. Of course, these investigative and therapeutic measures are costly and often out of reach of people with schizophrenia, in which case local advocacy is required.

How does having schizophrenia affect sexual function and sexual health?

Sexual function is a normal part of human activity and an important part of interpersonal relationships. There are many ways in which sexual function can be compromised in people with psychosis. First of all, there is a clear social impact of having a diagnosis of schizophrenia. While much of this may be related to stigma, a large proportion is internal, in the sense that schizophrenia can affect people's ability to interact socially and reduce their self-confidence in establishing sexual relationships.

Core sexual physiology may, just as in the general population, be impaired for various reasons, including age, tobacco smoking, obesity, diabetes, vascular disease, sedentary lifestyles, and alcohol use. Even during a first episode of psychosis, sexual dysfunction is common, and interestingly it is even evident in a substantial portion of people with prodromal psychotic symptoms who have never received antipsychotic medication (Marques et al., 2012).

Medications used to treat psychosis can affect sexual function in many different ways. Libido can be directly affected by changes in dopamine or indirectly by side effects such as sedation. Peripheral autonomic effects can interfere with sexual physiology, while whole-body side effects such as diabetes or dyslipidaemias can affect sexual function in the longer term. Comorbid conditions such as depression and anxiety can also compromise sexual function, just as they do in the general population. The relationship between medications and sexual function is discussed in Chapter 6, but it is important to note here how important and immediate this problem is to patients. The UK mental health charity, Rethink Mental Illness, conducted a survey of 2475 people as part of The Schizophrenia Commission (Rethink Mental Illness, 2012). Sexual dysfunction was ranked as one of the most troublesome antipsychotic side effects. It is also a common reason for medication non-adherence.

Enquiry about sexual function is important. Sensitive questioning is required, covering the domains shown in Fig. 4.2 and Fig. 4.3. Where problems are identified, it is important to recognize and treat any underlying causes and provide lifestyle advice, weight reduction and exercise strategies, as well as smoking cessation assistance (see Chapters 5, 8, and 9). Depression should be treated where appropriate, with care not to exacerbate sexual problems by prescription of

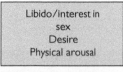

Libido/interest in
sex
Desire
Physical arousal

Masturbation
Frequency
Attitude

Orgasm/ejaculation
Frequency
Pain
Ease of orgasm/ejaculation

Men
Frequency/quality of erections
Timing of ejaculation
Fluid ejaculated

Women
Physical response to sexual
arousal
Satisfaction with sexual life

Satisfaction with sexual
life

Fig. 4.2 Areas to enquire about in sexual function history.

Data from *British Journal of Psychiatry*, 181, 2002, Smith SM, O'Keane V, Murray RM, 'Sexual dysfunction in patients taking conventional antipsychotic medication', The Royal College of Psychiatrists.

antidepressants that themselves carry sexual side effects. If antipsychotic medication seems to be a major contributor to sexual problems, a careful discussion should be facilitated with the patient (and their partner, where desired) regarding possible switching of agents. Phosphodiesterase inhibitors can be helpful, although care needs to be taken if the individual is at cardiovascular risk. They are also costly.

A related topic is sexual health. Rates of blood-borne diseases are elevated in people with psychosis. Furthermore, when someone is less well, behavioural impulsivity and disorganization can make life more chaotic, leading to a risk of sexually transmitted infections or unplanned pregnancies. Clear discussion of contraceptive needs and safe sex advice is an important part of the management plan of someone with a psychotic illness.

Pt. No. ____ Date. ____	
Each statement is followed by a TRUE or FALSE answer. Read each statement carefully and decide which response best describes how you feel. Then put a circle round the corresponding response. If you are not completely sure which response is more accurate, circle the response that you feel is most appropriate. Please ask the person interviewing you if there are any words you do not understand. Do not spend too long on each statement. It is important that you answer each question as honestly as possible. Remember to answer every question.	
ALL INFORMATION WILL BE TREATED WITH THE STRICTEST CONFIDENCE.	
Over the past month	
1. I have thought about sex	
a. at least once per day	TRUE/FALSE
b. three times per week	TRUE/FALSE
c. less than once per week	TRUE/FALSE
d. less than once a fortnight	TRUE/FALSE
2. I never think about sex	TRUE/FALSE
3. I have found other people sexually desirable	TRUE/FALSE
4. I have not wanted to have sexual intercourse	TRUE/FALSE
5. I have enjoyed sex	TRUE/FALSE
6. I have not been particularly interested in sex	TRUE/FALSE
Over the past month	
7. I have been easily aroused sexually	TRUE/FALSE
8. It has taken longer than usual for me to become sexually aroused	TRUE/FALSE
9. I have been completely unable to become sexually aroused	TRUE/FALSE
10. Although I have been aroused mentally, nothing has happened physically	TRUE/FALSE
Please answer this next section only if you are male.	
Over the past month	
11. I have had erections (morning erections or erections on awaking)	
a. every day	TRUE/FALSE
b. about three times per week	TRUE/FALSE
c. less than once per week	TRUE/FALSE
d. less than once a fortnight	TRUE/FALSE
e. less than once per month	TRUE/FALSE

Fig. 4.3 The Sexual Function Questionnaire.

Reproduced from *British Journal of Psychiatry*, 181, Smith SM, O'Keane V, Murray RM, 'Sexual dysfunction in patients taking conventional antipsychotic medication', pp. 49-55. Copyright (2002) with permission of The Royal College of Psychiatrists.

12. I do not have erections	TRUE/FALSE
13. I am always able to achieve a full erection if I want to	TRUE/FALSE
14. I feel that my erections are not as full now as they used to be	TRUE/FALSE
15. I am never able to achieve a full erection	TRUE/FALSE
16. I rarely achieve a full erection	TRUE/FALSE
17. Because I cannot achieve a full erection, I am unable to have intercourse	TRUE/FALSE
Please answer this next section only if you are female	
Over the past month	
18. Sex has been difficult or painful for me because I do not respond physically as I ought to	TRUE/FALSE
19. My physical response to sexual stimulation is different now to what it used to be	TRUE/FALSE
20. My physical response to sexual stimulation is better now than it used to be	TRUE/FALSE
21. My physical response to sexual stimulation is worse now than it used to be	TRUE/FALSE
Over the past month	
22. I have masturbated	
a. at least once a day	TRUE/FALSE
b. about three times per week	TRUE/FALSE
c. about once per week	TRUE/FALSE
d. less than once per fortnight	TRUE/FALSE
e. less than once per month	TRUE/FALSE
23. I feel that masturbation is wrong	TRUE/FALSE
24. I never masturbate	TRUE/FALSE
25. I rarely masturbate	TRUE/FALSE
26. I have masturbated more often than I usually do	TRUE/FALSE
27. I have masturbated less than I usually do	TRUE/FALSE
Over the past month	
28. I have not achieved orgasm/ejaculation by any means at all	TRUE/FALSE
29. I have had orgasms/ejaculations as often as I have wanted	TRUE/FALSE
30. I have never had an orgasm/ejaculation	TRUE/FALSE
31. Orgasm/ejaculation has been painful for me	TRUE/FALSE
32. My orgasm/ejaculation has been different to before	TRUE/FALSE
33. I have an orgasm/ejaculate every time I have sex/masturbate	TRUE/FALSE

Fig. 4.3 Continued

Please answer the following if you are male	
34. I ejaculate a long time after I have achieved orgasm	TRUE/FALSE
35. My ejaculation happens too quickly	TRUE/FALSE
36. The amount of fluid that I produce when I ejaculate is less than I used to produce before	TRUE/FALSE
37. The amount of fluid that I produce when I ejaculate is more than I used to produce before	TRUE/FALSE
38. The colour of the fluid that I produce when I ejaculate is different to before	TRUE/FALSE
Instructions for Interviewer	
A. Although this has the appearance of a structured questionnaire, the nature of the topic often means that you will need to clarify terms in order to ensure that the subjects know what is being asked of them. Also, if you are able to talk about sex, the subjects may feel more comfortable when filling in the questionnaire.	
B. Remind the subjects that the questions are quite personal, but also normalise the experience by reminding them of the usual process of sexual intercourse and the problems that people might encounter if their sexual function is poor (e.g. "Usually in order for people to have sex, they have to have an erection, some people find that they have difficulties with this. Section three asks questions about this area" or "Some people complain of difficulties with their sex life, they may have problems getting aroused sexually or they can't have orgasms, this questionnaire asks about this kind of thing").	
C. Section Two: sexual arousal involves the mental phenomena of being sexually interested and is usually accompanied by penile erection in males and vaginal lubrication and swelling of the vaginal walls in females (usual physical response after sexual stimulation in women).	
D. Terms	
Erection — when the penis gets hard or stiff.	
Vaginal lubrication — when the vagina becomes moist.	
Orgasm — the feeling that happens at the end of sex. This is usually accompanied by overwhelming physical sensations in women, along with vaginal wall contractions. In men it is accompanied by ejaculation.	
Ejaculation — the production of seminal fluid or semen.	

Fig. 4.3 Continued

What about oral health?

The teeth and mouth are often neglected areas when caring for people with schizophrenia. Oral health is poor in this group and impacts quality of life, social functioning, and self-esteem and can add to stigma. Additionally, gum disease is associated with a risk of cardiovascular disease. Moore et al. (2015) reviewed the literature on this topic and reported that people with severe mental illness are more likely to have lost all their teeth or to have decayed, missing, and filled teeth than are the

Table 4.2 Summary of poor oral health in schizophrenia	
Problems	Dry mouth (xerostomia) Missing teeth Edentulism Dental caries Excess fillings Dental abscess Periodontal disease
Causes	Inadequate oral hygiene Fewer dental check-ups Smoking Poor diet with high sugar intake Reduced personal perception of dental need Inflexibility of dental teams
Associations	Greater risk of cardiovascular disease Reduced quality of life Diminished social functioning Effects on self-esteem.
Management	Enhance awareness of oral health issues in mental health staff Education for patients Provide toothbrushes and fluoridated toothpastes in hospital Support registration with a local dentist More frequent dental visits Support to achieve good plaque control Consideration of fluoride varnishes and high-fluoride toothpastes Good communication between mental health and dental teams Flexible appointment times and duration Management of dental anxiety Smoking cessation advice Advice on alcohol, diet, and oral hygiene

Data from *Acta Psychiatrica Scandinavica*, 11, 2015, Moore S, Daly B, Shiers D et al, 'Promoting physical health by reducing disparities in medical and dental care'.

general population (see Table 4.2). Poor oral hygiene is likely to contribute to this; people with schizophrenia brush their teeth less often than the general population and are exposed to other risk factors such as smoking, xerostomia as a side effect of medication, and poor diet with a high sugar intake, especially from carbonated drinks. On top of this, people may fail to realize that they need dental care, while on the flip-side, dental care may not be adequately available, flexible, or affordable.

Solutions include enhanced awareness of oral health among mental health clinicians and service providers, plus education for patients. Providing toothbrushes and fluoridated toothpaste on admission to inpatient units and supporting registration with local dentists may help. As people with schizophrenia are at high risk of both tooth decay and periodontal disease, it is suggested that that they should attend the dentist more frequently than the general population (Moore et al., 2015). Flexible approaches to dental appointment times and duration, as well as active management of dental anxiety and general health promotion regarding smoking, alcohol use, diet, and dental hygiene, are also recommended.

Cancer deaths are higher in people with schizophrenia: but is cancer more common?

There is some inconsistency in the literature regarding cancer risks among people with schizophrenia. A large study in Taiwan over 9 years found that those with schizophrenia were 29% less likely than the general population to develop cancer, although mortality from cancer was a third higher (Chou et al., 2011). This reinforces data from a number of other jurisdictions that it is the discrepancy between rates of cancer and rates of death from cancer that is most important. Again, this is an indicator of the suboptimal care people with schizophrenia all too often receive (see Chapter 2).

There are various theories as to why people with schizophrenia who develop cancers tend to have worse outcomes compared to the general population. Uptake of screening for cancer is lower. For example, women with severe mental illnesses such as schizophrenia are less likely to receive breast and cervical cancer screening than those without a major mental illness (Woodhead et al., 2016). It has been thought that the poorer outcomes were as a result of people with schizophrenia presenting later in the course of their illness, but a recent study in London reported no differences in staging at the time of presentation. There was still poorer survival than in controls, suggesting that there are problems with access to treatment post diagnosis rather than simply late diagnosis (Chang et al., 2014). In keeping with this theory, Kisley et al. (2013) found that people with schizophrenia who developed cancer received, on average, fewer sessions of chemotherapy and were less likely to receive radiotherapy or surgical intervention.

Breast cancer is particularly important to mention in this context—there have long been worries of an increased risk of breast cancer in female patients with schizophrenia. The concern arises in part because of a proposed influence of prolactin on mammary carcinogenesis (see Chapter 6). The literature on the prevalence of breast cancer in female patients with schizophrenia is mixed, and the conclusions that can be drawn from prospective studies are limited, with a wide range of risk ratios for both pre- and post-menopausal women. There is therefore no conclusive evidence that antipsychotic medications increase the risk of breast malignancy and mortality. It is likely that other risk factors such as nulliparity, as well as obesity, diabetes, and lifestyle choices, such as alcohol use and smoking, probably are of more relevance in individual breast cancer cases (De Hert et al., 2016). Clearly women with schizophrenia should be supported to attend routine breast screening programmes and assisted with informed decision-making should any aberrant lesions be detected.

Do we ask about pain?

One-third of patients with schizophrenia report pain on questioning and this is linked to quality of life (Stubbs et al., 2015a). Yet pain is rarely enquired about in clinical practice. Many physical health disorders have pain as their first presentation. It may therefore be relevant that people with schizophrenia have decreased pain sensitivity and a higher pain threshold and tolerance compared to controls (Stubbs et al., 2015c). While it is possible that these differences in pain perception and tolerance in schizophrenia may influence health-seeking behaviours, it is no excuse for not asking about and effectively managing pain syndromes in people with schizophrenia.

Is surgery a more straightforward area in people with schizophrenia?

It appears not. A report on the outcomes of appendicitis surgery in people with psychosis found that although people with schizophrenia reported symptoms at around the same time as everybody else, when the surgical intervention itself took place, the natural course of the illness was more advanced; 80% of people had advanced appendicitis or perforated or gangrenous appendices at the time of surgery (Cooke et al., 2007). Unsurprisingly, therefore, morbidity and mortality rates were much higher in patients with schizophrenia than in the comparator group (Cooke et al., 2007). It is interesting to speculate as to whether this difference relates to the alterations in pain thresholds described.

Conclusion

People with schizophrenia are at high risk of developing many physical health conditions. Even when the risk of developing a particular health condition is no higher than in the general population, outcomes are generally worse. This is likely to relate to difficulties in accessing care in a timely fashion. Some of this may be due to impediments in recognizing that there is a problem, perhaps as a result of altered pain sensitivity. The disorganization dimension of psychosis and cognitive problems may mean that setting up appointments with healthcare professionals may be a challenge without support. Disorganization and cognitive and motivational difficulties may make complex treatment regimens difficult to put into practice. Much work is needed to allow healthcare professionals across all disciplines to make reasonable adjustments to provide equity in the physical healthcare of people with psychotic illnesses.

REFERENCES

Benros M, Eaton W, Mortensen PB (2014). The epidemiologic evidence linking autoimmune diseases and psychosis. *Biological Psychiatry* 75, 300–306.

Chang CK, Hayes RD, Broadbent MT, Hotopf M, Davies E, Møller H, Stewart R (2014). A cohort study on mental disorders, stage of cancer at diagnosis and subsequent survival. *BMJ Open* 29, 4.

Chou FH, Tsai KY, Su CY, Lee CC (2011). The incidence and relative risk factors for developing cancer among patients with schizophrenia: a nine-year follow-up study. *Schizophrenia Research* 129, 97–103.

Cooke BK, Magas LT, Virgo KS, Feinberg B, Adityanjee A, Johnson FE (2007). Appendectomy for appendicitis in patients with schizophrenia. *American Journal of Surgery* 193, 41–48.

Crews M, Lally J, Gardner-Sood, P, Howes O, Smith S, Murray RM, et al. (2013). Vitamin D deficiency in first episode psychosis: case–control study. *Schizophrenia Research* 150, 533–537.

De Hert M, Peuskens J, Sabbe T, Mitchell AJ, Stubbs B, Neven P, et al. (2016). Relationship between prolactin, breast cancer risk, and antipsychotics in patients with schizophrenia: a critical review. *Acta Psychiatrica Scandinavica* 133, 5–22.

Gomez L, Stubbs B, Shirazi A, Vancampfort D, Gaughran F, Lally J (2016). Lower bone mineral density at the hip and lumbar spine in people with psychosis versus controls: a comprehensive review and skeletal site-specific meta-analysis. *Current Osteoporosis Reports* 14, 249–259.

Kisely S, Crowe E, Lawrence D (2013). Cancer-related mortality in people with mental illness. *JAMA Psychiatry* 70, 209–217.

Marques TR, Smith L, Bonaccorso S, Gaughran F, Kolliakou A, Dazzan P, et al. (2012). Sexual dysfunction in people with prodromal signs of psychosis and in the first psychotic episode. *British Journal of Psychiatry* 201, 131–136.

McGrath JJ, Eyles DW, Pedersen CB, Anderson C, Ko P, Burne TH, et al. (2010). Neonatal vitamin D status and risk of schizophrenia: a population-based case-control study. *Archives of General Psychiatry* 67, 889–894.

Moore S, Daly B, Shiers D, Mitchell A, Gaughran F (2015). Promoting physical health by reducing disparities in medical and dental care. *Acta Psychiatrica Scandinavica* 132, 109–121.

Mors O, Mortensen PB, Ewald H (1999). A population-based register study of the association between schizophrenia and rheumatoid arthritis. *Schizophrenia Research* 40, 67–74.

Olfson M, Gerhard T, Huang C, Crystal S, Stroup TS (2015). Premature mortality among adults with schizophrenia in the United States. *JAMA Psychiatry* 72, 1172–1181.

Rethink Mental Illness (2012). *The Abandoned Illness: A Report by the Schizophrenia Commission*. London: Rethink Mental Illness. https://www.rethink.org/media/514093/TSC_main_report_14_nov.pdf

Sharan P (2017). Perspectives from resource poor settings. *World Psychiatry* 16, 42–43.

Smith SM, O'Keane V, Murray RM (2002). Sexual dysfunction in patients taking conventional antipsychotic medication. *British Journal of Psychiatry* 181, 49–55.

Stubbs B, Gardner-Sood P, Smith S, Ismail K, Greenwood K, Patel A, et al. (2015a). Pain is independently associated with reduced health related quality of life in people with psychosis. *Psychiatry Research* 15, 585–591.

Stubbs B, Gaughran F, Mitchell AJ, De Hert M, Farmer R, Soundy A, et al. (2015b). Schizophrenia and the risk of fractures: a systematic review and comparative meta-analysis. *General Hospital Psychiatry* 37, 126–133.

Stubbs B, Thompson T, Acaster S, Vancampfort D, Gaughran F, Correll CU (2015c). Decreased pain sensitivity among people with schizophrenia: a meta-analysis of experimental pain induction studies. *Pain* 156, 2121–2131.

Stubbs B, Koyanagi A, Veronese N, Vancampfort D, Solmi M, Gaughran F, et al. (2016a). Physical multimorbidity and psychosis: comprehensive cross sectional analysis including 242,952 people across 48 low and middle-income countries. *BMC Medicine* 14, 189.

Stubbs B, Vancampfort D, Veronese N, Solmi M, Gaughran F, Manu P, et al. (2016b). The prevalence and predictors of obstructive sleep apnea in major depressive disorder, bipolar disorder and schizophrenia: a systematic review and meta-analysis. *Journal of Affective Disorders* 197, 259–267.

Wang MT, Tsai CL, Lin CW, Yeh CB, Wang YH, Lin HL (2017). Association between antipsychotic agents and risk of acute respiratory failure in patients with chronic obstructive pulmonary disease. *JAMA Psychiatry* 74, 252–260.

Woodhead C, Cunningham R, Ashworth M, Barley E, Stewart RJ, Henderson MJ (2016). Cervical and breast cancer screening uptake among women with serious mental illness: a data linkage study. *BMC Cancer* 21, 819.

CHAPTER 4

Smoking and schizophrenia

KEY POINTS
• Cigarette smoking is highly prevalent among people with schizophrenia.
• Reasons for such high rates are multifactorial and encompass neurobiological and psychosocial parameters.
• Quit rates among people with schizophrenia are generally low and reinstatement common.
• Clinicians should ensure they ask their patients about smoking and assist them in quitting and remaining abstinent.

That cigarette smoking is very common in people with schizophrenia is a robust finding from numerous diverse jurisdictions across the globe. Furthermore, the rates seem not to have fallen substantially despite a reduction in most countries in rates of smoking in the general population. This is shown starkly in Australia, where public health campaigns and high costs of cigarettes have contributed to a marked reduction in cigarette consumption in the general population: in 2010 the rate was 19%. In contrast, in the 2010 Study of High Impact Psychoses (SHIP), a representative sample of people in treatment for psychotic disorders, 70% of those participants with schizophrenia were smokers (Cooper et al., 2012). There had been practically no reduction in smoking rates over the 12 years since the first Australian National Survey of psychotic disorders. Similar discrepancies between general population smoking rates and rates in people with schizophrenia can be seen from data from the US (see Evins et al., 2015) and other countries (de Leon and Diaz, 2005).

Not only do people with schizophrenia smoke at high rates, they also smoke a great deal. In the SHIP study, average daily consumption was 20.8 cigarettes per day. There were high rates of severe dependence, with 60% having their first cigarette within 5 minutes of waking and a mean Fagerström Test for Nicotine Dependence rating of 5.9, indicative of high dependence (Table 5.1). It has been shown in other studies that people with schizophrenia can extract nicotine highly efficiently from a cigarette, adding to their additional risk of high dependence.

Table 5.1 The Fagerström Test for Nicotine Dependence		
PLEASE TICK (√) ONE BOX FOR EACH QUSTION		
How soon after waking do you smoke your first cigarette?	Within 5 minutes	☐ 1
	5–30 minutes	☐ 2
	31–60 minutes	☐ 3
Do you find it difficult to refrain from smoking in places where it is forbidden (e.g. church, library)?	Yes	☐ 1
	No	☐ 0
Which cigarette would you hate to give up?	First thing in the morning	☐ 1
	Any other	☐ 0
How many cigarettes a day do you smoke?	10 or less	☐ 0
	11–20	☐ 1
	21–30	☐ 2
	31 or more	☐ 3
Do you smoke more frequently in the morning?	Yes	☐ 1
	No	☐ 0
Do you smoke even if you are sick in bed most of the day?	Yes	☐ 1
	No	☐ 0
	Total score	

SCORE   1–2 = low dependence   5–7 = moderate dependence
            3–4 = low to moderate dependence   8+ = high dependence

Reproduced from Heatherton TF, Kozlowski LT, Frecker RC et al., 'The Fagerström Test for Nicotine Dependence: a revision of the Fagerström Tolerance Questionnaire', *British Journal of Addiction*, 86, pp. 1119–1127. Copyright (1991) K. O. Fagerström. Please note that since publication the test has been renamed the Fagerstrom Test for Cigarette Dependence (FTCD)

Why do people with schizophrenia smoke?

Reasons for smoking among people with schizophrenia include social affiliation, in that so many of their peers smoke and until recently cigarettes were part of the culture of many psychiatric institutions. Boredom is also often cited as a reason for smoking among people with schizophrenia. And of course nicotine is highly addictive, hence, once started it is difficult to stop smoking. Galazyn et al. (2010) reported that smokers with schizophrenia were, compared to non-psychiatric controls, more likely to endorse the following as reasons for smoking: stimulation (as with other drugs such as amphetamines), amelioration of negative affect, and avoidance of nicotine withdrawal.

It is clear that neurobiological factors play a role in the high rates of smoking among people with schizophrenia. Nicotine releases dopamine, the 'reward' monoamine, and there is a relative deficit of dopamine in mesocortical projections in people with schizophrenia, expressly subsuming negative and cognitive deficits (George et al., 2003). Nicotine also has cognitive-enhancing properties. Thus, some of the neurocognitive deficits seen in some people with schizophrenia (such as attention, memory, and verbal learning) can be ameliorated (in the short term at least) by nicotine (George et al., 2002).

It is puzzling that public health messages and cost increases that have been so effective in reducing rates of smoking in many countries have not had any meaningful impact in people with schizophrenia. Studies have tried to understand how people with schizophrenia view smoking cessation. Kelly et al. (2012) showed that smokers with schizophrenia were less likely than smokers without schizophrenia to be aware of the negative health consequences of smoking but more likely to embrace social motivations to quit. Contrary to popular belief, many smokers with schizophrenia do wish to quit and many attempt quitting, but relapse rates are very high. For example, in the SHIP study, 72% of smokers had tried to quit a mean of 4.5 times (Cooper et al., 2012).

Can smoking cause schizophrenia?

There has been recent interest as to whether smoking can increase the risk of developing schizophrenia. General population studies have found tobacco consumption to be associated with certain psychosis-like experiences and long-term cohort studies have shown an association between cigarette smoking and the later manifestation of psychotic symptoms (McGrath et al., 2016). A Swedish study (Kendler et al., 2015) used a clever co-relative design to investigate this further. These investigators found that light smoking was associated with an increased hazard of schizophrenia, with a hazard ratio (HR) of 2.21 (95% CI, 1.90–2.56) for women and 2.15 (95% CI, 1.25–3.44) for men. For heavy smoking, the hazards were even higher: a HR of 3.45 (95% CI, 2.95–4.03) for females and 3.80 (95% CI, 1.19–6.60) for males. This suggests a dose–response effect which strengthens the case for a causal association. Kendler et al. (2015) also performed sophisticated modelling that allowed them to estimate that the association could not be explained simply by genetic factors relevant to both schizophrenia and smoking. Thus, for monozygotic twins, heavy smoking was associated with a HR of 1.69 (95% CI, 1.17–2.44) suggesting an independent effect of smoking.

What are the physical health risks associated with smoking?

The health risks of cigarette smoking are well described. In people with schizophrenia, there are particular risks associated with this behaviour as generally their physical health is often suboptimal and the general healthcare they receive is all too often lacking or at least not as assertive as in people without schizophrenia (see Chapter 4). It is thus surprising that rates of lung cancer are not markedly in excess among people with schizophrenia. Possible explanations include people dying of other causes (notably cardiovascular) at such high rates and so relatively young that they do not attain the age at which cancer would be most likely to manifest. There is also the well-established fact, as outlined elsewhere in this book, that there is a health inequality when it comes to people with schizophrenia and thus cancers might be missed and/or undertreated in people with schizophrenia.

But the main physical health risk associated with tobacco consumption is that it contributes additively to the risk of cardiovascular events. As detailed in Chapter 3 of this book, people with schizophrenia are at heightened risk, compared to the general population, of a range of cardiovascular risk factors. Tobacco smoking is arguably the most important single reversible cause of early cardiovascular death among people with schizophrenia and is thus a major public health concern.

What can be done to address smoking in people with schizophrenia?

Despite the failure of public health messages to impact overall smoking rates among people with schizophrenia, it is important that public health initiatives are continued. But it is also clear that such messaging needs to be responsive specifically to the needs and attitudes of people with schizophrenia and targeted through mental health and other clinics. Also, it is imperative that clinicians who have contact with people with schizophrenia enquire about cigarette smoking in order to offer help and assistance in harm reduction and eventual quitting.

Establishing people's understanding of the health risks associated with smoking at an individual level, and trying to motivate them to quit, should be part of every mental health clinician's skill set. Establishing the extent of smoking (i.e. number of cigarettes smoked per day) and the degree of dependence is an important start. A reasonably quick and validated approach is to use the Fagerström Test (Table 5.1) but if this is not feasible to use in its entirety, the specific items on quantity smoked and how soon after waking the individual has their first cigarette, are adequate. Offering smoking cessation advice, outlining the methods available, and referral to quitlines and/or to a health professional particularly skilled in smoking cessation, should be routine. This is summarized in an algorithm dubbed the 'five As' (Ask, Advise, Assess, Assist, Arrange (Fig. 5.1).

Smoking cessation trials in people with schizophrenia have generally incorporated, at the least, behavioural smoking cessation techniques: these have been reviewed by Evins et al. (2015) and are summarized in Box 5.1. Other studies have included other healthy lifestyle elements, targeting diet and exercise: these approaches are outlined in Chapters 9 and 10 of this book.

CHAPTER 5

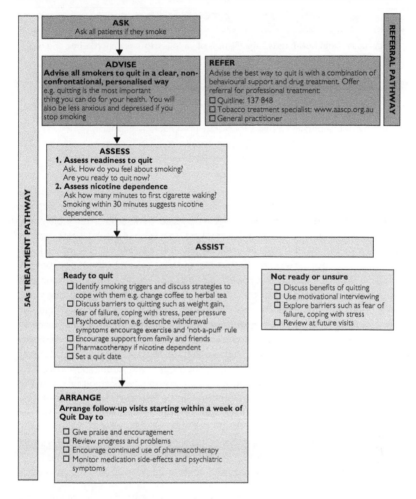

Fig. 5.1 Combined 5As and referral pathway for smoking cessation.

Reproduced from Mendelsohn CP, Kirby DP, Castle DJ, 'Smoking and mental illness. An update for psychiatrists', *Australasian Psychiatry*, 23, 1, pp. 37–45. Copyright (2015) SAGE Publications.

What medications are available to assist smoking cessation?

Pharmacotherapy can play a key part in helping people stop smoking. In many jurisdictions, nicotine replacement therapy (NRT), bupropion, and varenicline have approved indications for smoking cessation, in conjunction with a psychological intervention (Table 5.2). Evins et al. (2015) conducted a systematic review

> **Box 5.1** Summary of behavioural smoking cessation techniques
>
> ● *Education* about health risks, effectiveness of various treatment approaches, and relationship between smoking and psychiatric symptoms.
> ● *Motivational enhancement*, including establishing motivational stage and helping weigh risks and benefits of continuing smoking versus quitting.
> ● *Cognitive behavioural strategies* including identification of situations in which smoking is likely to occur and specific triggers; development of coping strategies, notably for high-risk situations; and planning for relapse prevention.
>
> Data from *Harvard Review of Psychiatry*, 23, 2015, Evins AE, Cather C, Laffer A, 'Treatment of tobacco use disorders in smokers with serious mental illness: towards clinical best practice', Wolters Kluwer Health.

of the use of such agents in people with schizophrenia and related disorders and concluded that they are effective and generally safe; they summarize: 'Converging evidence indicates that a majority of smokers with serious mental illness want to quit smoking and that available pharmacotherapeutic cessation aids combined with behavioural support are both effective for and well tolerated by these smokers' (p. 90). It is as well to add that people with mental illnesses such as schizophrenia need extra monitoring when commencing such agents, due to their often high levels of nicotine dependence; their often being on medications that might interact with chemicals in tobacco or cigarette paper (e.g. induction of enzymes involved in the metabolism of clozapine and olanzapine); and their increased vulnerability to psychiatric symptoms including those which can be exacerbated when stopping smoking and/or have been associated with bupropion and varenicline in particular.

NRT is the most well studied and widely employed pharmacological adjunct to smoking cessation. NRT is available in numerous forms, including patches, lozenges, gum, and inhalant forms. In people smoking more than 10 cigarettes per day, a full-strength patch (21 mg for 24 hours) should be used. It is not uncommon for people with heavy dependence (as is so common among smokers with schizophrenia) to use additional forms of NRT as well as the patch. Some find it difficult to cease smoking altogether and need to be warned not to smoke while the patch is *in situ*.

There is also evidence that NRT can be helpful in reducing aggression in acute settings. For example, Allen et al. (2011) conducted a placebo-controlled trial of NRT patches in an emergency department setting in the US and found that active NRT reduced rates of aggression in people with mental illnesses such as schizophrenia. It would seem sensible to offer NRT to smokers with mental illness who are not allowed to continue their habit in a hospital setting.

Bupropion is an antidepressant which blocks the reuptake of noradrenaline and dopamine and also acts as an antagonist at the nicotinic acetylcholinergic receptor. For smoking cessation, it is used in a dose of 150 mg per day for 3 days, then 150 mg twice a day. A course of 9 weeks is advised, with smoking cessation planned for around a week after commencement. There is a risk of precipitation of

Table 5.2 Approved drugs for treating nicotine dependence

Drug	Recommended dose	Course of treatment	Common adverse effects	Directions for use
Nicotine replacement therapies (NRTs)				
Nicotine patch 24 h: 21 mg, 14 mg, 7 mg 16 h: 25 mg, 10 mg	Start with full-strength patch if ≥ 10 cigarettes/day	12 weeks	Insomnia, disturbed dreams (24 h patch) Skin irritation	Apply in the morning to upper arm, chest, or back and rotate application site daily
Nicotine mouth spray 1 mg per spray	1–2 sprays every 30–60 min Maximum 4 sprays/hour or 64 sprays/day	12 weeks	Mouth/throat irritation, nausea, dyspepsia, headache, hiccups	Fast-acting craving relief. Spray under tongue or onto inside of cheek
Nicotine oral strips 2.5 mg	Initially 1 strip every 1–2 h, up to 15/day	12 weeks	Nausea, throat irritation, hiccups, headache	Fast-acting craving relief for less dependent smokers. Place on tongue and apply to palate: dissolves in 2–3 min
Nicotine lozenges 2 mg, 4 mg	2 mg and 4 mg 9–15/day	12 weeks	Nausea, hiccups, heartburn, flatulence	Allow to dissolve in the mouth over 20–30 min, moving around from time to time
Nicotine mini lozenges 1.5 mg, 4 mg	1.5 mg: 9–20 times/day 4 mg: 9–15/day	12 weeks	Nausea, hiccups, heartburn, flatulence	Allow to dissolve in the mouth over 10–15 min, moving around from time to time
Nicotine gum 2 mg, 4 mg	2 mg: 8–20/day 4 mg: 4–10/day Use 4 mg if TTFC[a] ≤30 min	12 weeks	Hiccups, nausea, jaw discomfort, mouth/throat irritation	Instruct patients 'on park and chew' technique.[b] Avoid in people with dentures
Nicotine inhalator 15 mg per cartridge	3–6 cartridges per day	12 weeks	Cough, mouth/throat irritation, nausea	Frequent shallow puffs. Satisfies hand-to-mouth habit

(*Continued*)

Table 5.2 Continued

Drug	Recommended dose	Course of treatment	Common adverse effects	Comments
Non-nicotine tablets				
Varenicline 0.5 mg, 1 mg	0.5 mg/day for 3 days, then 0.5 twice daily for 4 days, then 1 mg twice daily	12 weeks; optional second course	Nausea, insomnia, disturbed dreams, headache, drowsiness	Most effective monotherapy. Take with a meal to reduce nausea. No known drug interactions. Contraindicated in pregnancy and lactation
Bupropion 150 mg	150 mg/day for 3 days, then 150 mg twice daily	9 weeks	Seizure risk 1:1000, insomnia, headache, dry mouth	Elevated seizure risk. Numerous potential drug interactions. Contraindicated in pregnancy, lactation

[a] TTFC: time to first cigarette.

[b] Chew gum slowly until peppery taste appears and then place gum in the buccal pouch until taste fades. Chew again until taste appears. Repeat cycle for 30 min then discard. Avoid swallowing nicotine.

Reproduced from Mendelsohn CP, Kirby DP, Castle DJ, 'Smoking and mental illness. An update for psychiatrists', *Australasian Psychiatry*, 23, 1, pp. 37–45. Copyright (2015) SAGE Publications.

hypomania or mania in those with a bipolar predisposition, albeit it is often used as a treatment for bipolar depression, along with a mood stabilizer. A particular issue with bupropion is a 1 in 1000 risk of seizures and it is relatively contraindicated in individuals with a history of seizures, head trauma, eating disorders, or alcohol dependence. Bupropion inhibits cytochrome P450-2D6 and thus interacts with some serotonergic and tricyclic antidepressants and certain antipsychotics. It should not be used in conjunction with monoamine oxidase inhibitors.

Varenicline is a partial agonist at the nicotinic acetylcholinergic receptor and also acts as an antagonist at that receptor, thus reducing the rewarding effects of nicotine. It is a highly effective smoking cessation agent and has proven superior to NRT and bupropion as monotherapy, with up to three times the cessation rate. An incremental dose schedule is recommended, commencing at 0.5 mg per day for 3 days, then 0.5 mg twice a day for 4 days, then 1 mg twice a day for the remainder of the 12-week course. An additional 12 weeks is often helpful in consolidation of smoking cessation, expressly in people with heavy dependence as is so often the case in smokers with schizophrenia. Varenicline can cause nausea but this is reduced if it is taken with food. A particular concern regarding varenicline has been a series of reports of significant effects on mood, and suicidality in particular, in people taking varenicline. A number of studies have explored the relevant literature, including using meta-analytic techniques, and these have generally failed to support a causal association between varenicline and depression and suicide (Gibbons and Mann, 2013). Also, studies specifically of people with mood and psychotic disorders have shown it can be a safe and effective agent in these clinical groups (Williams et al., 2012).

The neuropsychiatric safety of the various smoking cessation medications has been recently demonstrated in a large-scale, double-blind randomized controlled trial labelled EAGLES (Anthenelli et al., 2016). EAGLES randomly assigned 8144 individuals—4116 of whom had an established mental illness—to receive either NRT (21 mg patch daily with taper), varenicline (2 mg daily), bupropion (300 mg daily), or placebo. There was a 12-week initial phase and a further 12-week follow-up. Varenicline was the most efficacious agent for smoking cessation and there was no statistical increase in neuropsychiatric side effects relative to the other study arms. While this study should make clinicians less concerned about adverse neuropsychiatric effects of varenicline in particular, careful counselling and monitoring is required to support those few individuals—with or without a psychiatric history—who do experience moderate or severe neuropsychiatric sequelae associated with any form of smoking cessation protocol.

In general, nicotine cessation is often associated with anxiety and mood effects as well as sleep disturbance. Warning people about these symptoms should be part of any comprehensive smoking cessation intervention and safety checks should be put in place such that any severe mood symptoms and/or suicidality are dealt with immediately.

It is also important to note that a number of psychotropic medications interact with smoking and adjustments might need to be made according to smoking status. These effects are summarized in Table 5.3.

Table 5.3 Clinically relevant psychotropic drug interactions with smoking

Class	Drug	Effect on smoking cessation	Clinical importance
Antipsychotics	Clozapine	Serum levels rise. Reduce dose by 50%	+++
	Olanzapine	Serum level rise. Reduce dose by 30%	+++
	Haloperidol	Serum levels may rise. Clinical	+
	Chlorpromazine	significance unclear	
	Fluphenazine		
Antidepressants	Fluvoxamine (SSRI)	Plasma levels may increase. May need dose reduction	++ +
	Duloxetine	Serum levels may rise. Clinical	+
	Mirtazapine	significance uncertain	+
	Imipramine	Serum levels may rise	
		Serum levels may rise. Monitor side effects	
Other drugs	Caffeine	Caffeine levels rise. Reduce caffeine by half within a week	+++
	Alcohol	Increased alcoholic levels, cognitive impairment, intoxication, sedation. Advise reduce alcohol intake	+++
	Benzodiazepines	Possible increased sedation due to loss of CNS stimulation by nicotine. May need lower dose	+
	Beta-blockers	Serum levels rise and effects enhanced. May need lower dose	+

Reproduced from Mendelsohn CP, Kirby DP, Castle DJ, 'Smoking and mental illness. An update for psychiatrists', *Australasian Psychiatry*, 23, 1, pp. 37–45. Copyright (2015) SAGE Publications.

What about e-cigarettes?

Electronic cigarettes (e-cigarettes) are battery-powered devices that release a vapour that can be inhaled. The vaporized liquid can contain nicotine and in this form e-cigarettes can substitute for cigarettes. The main virtue of this substitution is a much lower risk of those physical health problems that bedevil cigarette smoking (and which are largely due to the other constituents of tobacco and the paper in which it is wrapped): estimates place the physical health risk at some 5% of that associated with cigarettes. Other benefits include lower risk to others through passive smoking and also potentially more flexibility in 'dose reduction' as people move towards the ultimate aim of total cessation. Also, smoking-induced hepatic enzyme induction that enhances the metabolism of antipsychotics such as olanzapine and clozapine is not a factor with e-cigarettes and could allow lower doses of such drugs in smokers who switch (see Sharma et al., 2017).

The use of e-cigarettes and other such devices in people with schizophrenia has not been widely studied, but it seems a reasonable strategy for those who have failed other strategies. Objections to this approach include that it would go against consistent public health messages concerning smoking and that it might encourage people to take up smoking. These are legitimate concerns and have prevailed in certain jurisdictions where e-cigarettes are banned and prescription of the nicotine-containing fluids is not legally sanctioned. Further work is required to establish the place of e-cigarettes in helping people with schizophrenia to stop smoking.

Conclusion

Cigarette smoking is highly prevalent among people with schizophrenia. Reasons for such high rates are multifactorial and encompass neurobiological and psychosocial parameters. Quit rates among people with schizophrenia are generally low and reinstatement common. Clinicians should ensure they ask their patients about smoking; try to motivate them to quit; and offer behavioural/psychological and pharmacological interventions to assist them in quitting and remaining abstinent.

REFERENCES

Allen MH, Debanné M, Lazignac C, Adam E, Dickinson LM, Damsa C (2011). Effect of nicotine replacement therapy on agitation in smokers with schizophrenia: a double-blind, randomized, placebo-controlled study. American Journal of Psychiatry 186, 395–399.

Anthenelli RM, Benowitz NL, West R, St Aubin L, McRae T, Lawrence D, et al. (2016). Neuropsychiatric safety and efficacy of varenicline, bupropion, and nicotinic patch in smokers with and without psychiatric disorders (EAGLES): a double-blind, randomised, placebo-controlled clinical trial. Lancet 387, 2507–2520.

Cooper J, Mancuso SG, Borland R, Slade T, Galletly C, Castle D (2012). Tobacco smoking among people living with a psychotic illness: the Second Australian survey of Psychosis. Australian and New Zealand Journal of Psychiatry 46, 851–863.

De Leon J, Diaz FJ (2005). A meta-analysis of worldwide studies demonstrates an association between schizophrenia and tobacco smoking behaviours. Schizophrenia Research 76, 135–157.

Evins AE, Cather C, Laffer A (2015). Treatment of tobacco use disorders in smokers with serious mental illness: towards clinical best practice. Harvard Review of Psychiatry 23, 90–98.

George TP, Vessicchio JC, Termine A (2002). Effects of smoking abstinence on visuospatial working memory function in schizophrenia. Neuropsychopharmacology 26, 75–85.

George TP, Vessicchio JC, Termine A (2003). Nicotine and tobacco use in schizophrenia. In: Meyer JM, Nasrallah HA (eds) Medical Illness and Schizophrenia, pp. 81–98. Washington, DC: American Psychiatric Publishing, Inc.

Gibbons RD, Mann JJ (2013). Varenicline, smoking cessation and neuropsychiatric adverse events. *American Journal of Psychiatry* 170, 1460–1467.

Heatherton TF, Kozlowski LT, Frecker RC, Fagerstrom KO (1991). The Fagerström test for nicotine dependence: a revision of the Fagerstrom Tolerance Questionnaire. *British Journal of Addiction* 86, 1119–1127.

Kelly DL, Raley HG, Lo S, Wright K, Liu F, McMahon RP, et al. (2012). Perception of smoking risks and motivation to quit among nontreatment-seeking smokers with and without schizophrenia. *Schizophrenia Bulletin* 38, 543–551.

Kendler KS, Lönn SL, Sundquist J, Sundquist K (2015). Smoking and schizophrenia in population cohorts of Swedish women and men: a prospective co-relative control study. *American Journal of Psychiatry* 172, 1092–1100.

McGrath JJ, Alati R, Clavarino A, Williams GM, Bor W, Najman JM, et al. (2016). Age at first tobacco use and risk of subsequent psychosis-related outcomes: a birth cohort study. *Australian and New Zealand Journal of Psychiatry* 50, 577–583.

Mendelsohn CP, Kirby DP, Castle DJ (2015). Smoking and mental illness. An update for psychiatrists. *Australasian Psychiatry* 23, 37–43.

Sharma R, Gartner C, Castle DJ, Mendelsohn C (2017). Should we encourage smokers with severe mental illness to switch to electronic cigarettes? *Australian and New Zealand Journal of Psychiatry.* First Published March 8, 2017. DOI: 10.1177/0004867417697823

Williams JM, Anthenelli RM, Morris CD, Treadow J, Thompson JR, Yunis C, George TP (2012). A randomized, double-blind, placebo-controlled study evaluating the safety and efficacy of varenicline for smoking cessation in patients with schizophrenia or schizoaffective disorder. *Journal of Clinical Psychiatry* 73, 654–660.

CHAPTER 6

Effects of antipsychotic medications on physical health

KEY POINTS

- Antipsychotic medications are a key component of the treatment of schizophrenia and are often required long term.
- Individuals prescribed these medications often experience side effects and the management of these side effects is vital for quality of life.
- Side effects vary between drug classes, between individual drugs, and between patients.
- Prescribing requires thought and care and is reflected in shared decision-making processes.
- Where possible, prescribe medications that will not unduly add to long-term metabolic or other problems.

Antipsychotic medications are considered the cornerstone of the management of schizophrenia and related disorders. As these conditions are often enduring, antipsychotics are usually prescribed for long periods. Different medications are associated with different side effect profiles. The concept of grouping antipsychotics into classes is flawed but most commonly, we speak of 'typical' and 'atypical'—so termed because of their greater or lesser propensity to cause movement disorders. Typical and atypical antipsychotics are sometimes referred to as first- and second-generation agents, recognizing the evolution over time. In clinical practice, it is better to think of different medications as unique rather than simply being under the typical or atypical umbrella. Thus, each agent has a side effect profile that can be summarized as shown in Table 6.1. In this chapter, we focus mostly on the more modern antipsychotics as they tend to be most widely prescribed in clinical practice, at least in wealthy countries.

Large longitudinal studies such as the Clinical Antipsychotic Trials of Intervention Effectiveness (CATIE) (Lieberman et al., 2005) and Cost Utility of the Latest Antipsychotic Drugs in Schizophrenia Study (CUtLASS) (Jones et al., 2006) have shown that while the side effect profiles vary between typical and atypical antipsychotics, overall they can be equally difficult for the patient in terms of quality of life. At a more precise level, there are differences between individual drugs in their side effect profiles, largely related to the receptors targeted. Additionally, each person possesses a different constellation of the genes governing metabolism of medication; if someone breaks down a drug especially quickly they may need a higher dose

Table 6.1 Relative side effect profile of selected antipsychotics

Antipsychotic	Weight gain	ACh use	Prolactin	QTc prolongation	Sedation
Haloperidol	1	15	10	4	8
Chlorpromazine	11	13	5	N/A	13
Clozapine	13	1	N/A	N/A	15
Amisulpride	5	7	N/A	11	1
Olanzapine	15	3	4	6	10
Risperidone	8	11	11	7	7
Paliperidone	7	10	12	3	2
Zotepine	14	14	N/A	N/A	14
Quetiapine	10	4	2	5	11
Aripiprazole	4	5	1	2	5
Sertindole	9	2	9	12	3
Asenapine	6	9	3	8	9
Lurasidone	3	12	8	1	6
Iloperidone	12	6	6	9	4

ACh, anticholinergic agents, a proxy for extrapyramidal side effects; N/A, not applicable; QTc, QT interval, adjusted for cardiac rate.

Reproduced with permission from Castle D.J. and Buckley P.F., *Schizophrenia*, second edition, table 8.1, Copyright © 2015 with permission from Oxford University Press; data from *The Lancet*, 382, Leucht S, Cipriani A, Spineli L et al, Comparative efficacy and tolerability of 15 antipsychotic drugs in schizophrenia: a multiple-treatments meta-analysis, 951–962.

for therapeutic effect, or, if slow metabolizers, they may be particularly susceptible to side effects (Lally et al., 2016). Furthermore, taking a higher dose of medication, or combinations of different medications, can cause more side effects.

In this chapter, we outline the main physical health problems associated with the more commonly used antipsychotics. We commence with extrapyramidal effects, as the newer antipsychotics generally have a lower burden in this regard, but they can certainly still occur with these drugs and clinicians must be aware of the risks and be confident in assessing and treating them if they occur.

Are movement disorders on antipsychotics a thing of the past?

One of the major advantages touted for so-called atypical antipsychotics is their relatively (to typical agents) lower propensity to cause those acute and chronic extrapyramidal movement disorders that so bedevilled the use of medications such as haloperidol and trifluoperazine. In fact, such movement disorders can occur with all antipsychotics if the dose is high enough, with the possible exception of clozapine. This is because, until very recently, molecules in development were identified as potentially having antipsychotic activity if they were able to induce cataplexy in rats and thus likely to be a dopamine receptor antagonist. Unsurprisingly, therefore, every antipsychotic currently on the market antagonizes dopamine receptors postsynaptically. It thus remains vital that mental health clinicians have an understanding of the main dopaminergic tracts in the brain (Fig. 6.1) and appreciate the range of movement disorders associated with dopamine blockade. These disorders can be uncomfortable for the patient (e.g. akathisia), disfiguring (e.g. tardive dyskinesia) and sometimes prove fatal (e.g. acute laryngeal dystonias). Table 6.2 provides an overview of the various extrapyramidal movement disorders.

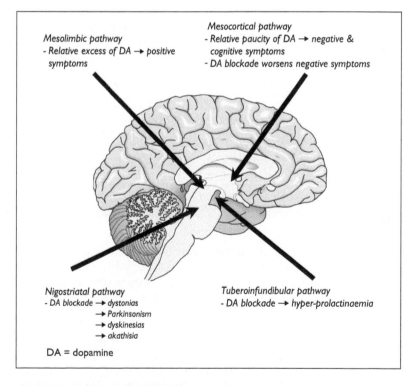

Fig. 6.1 The main dopaminergic tracts in the brain.

Reproduced with permission from Castle D.J. and Buckley P.F., *Schizophrenia*, second edition, figure 6.1, Copyright © 2015 with permission from Oxford University Press.

Table 6.2 Extrapyramidal movement disorders

		Signs and symptoms	Treatment
Parkinsonism		• Cogwheel rigidity • Shuffling gait with restricted arm swing • Restriction of affect ('mask like' facies)	• Lower dose of antipsychotic • Use atypical antipsychotic • Anticholinergic agent
Dystonias	Acute	• Opisthotonos • Laryngeal dystonia (can be fatal)	• Immediate treatment with anticholinergic (can use IMI or IVI if required)
	Tardive	• E.g. 'postural' abnormality with 'limping 'gait due to paraspinal muscle dystonia	• Lower dose • Use atypical agent • Anticholinergic agent
Dyskinesias	Acute		• Lower dose or change antipsychotic
	Tardive	• Oro-facio-bucco-lingual • Truncal and limb dyskinesias	• Complex: see text

Akathisia		• Observed motor restlessness
		• Subjective 'need to move', especially legs
			• Lower dose of antipsychotic
			• Use atypical antipsychotic
			• Cover with short-term:
			  o Beta-blocker
			  o Benzodiazepine
			  o Mirtazapine
			  o Clonidine

Reproduced with permission from Castle D.J. and Buckley P.F., *Schizophrenia*, second edition, table 8.3, Copyright © 2015 with permission from Oxford University Press.

Movement disorders derive from antagonism of the nigrostriatal dopaminergic pathways, causing extrapyramidal side effects (EPSEs). When managing movement disorders it is important to rate them systematically to allow assessment of change over time. There are well-established validated scales to facilitate this, but they tend to be too long to use in everyday clinical practice. A brief 'screen' for the main EPSEs is shown in Table 6.3.

The most dramatic movement side effect is *acute dystonia*, a rapid onset of painful and distressing muscle spasms. This occurs in about 10% of people prescribed antipsychotics, although mild cases are probably under-reported. It is more likely to manifest when people take antipsychotics for the first time, especially young males. Acute dystonia is usually not dangerous, unless it affects the laryngeal or pharyngeal muscles, but is upsetting and needs rapid

Table 6.3 A quick screen for extrapyramidal movement disorders

Ask the patient to:	Observe	Domain assessed
Walk freely then turn 180° and then return to observer	• Gait (e.g. stride, length, shuffling) • Turn (e.g. 'three-point' or taking extra steps) • Arm swing • Pill rolling tremor	Parkinsonism, paraspinal dystonias, abnormal involuntary movements
Hold arms out to side and then let them fall naturally	• How quickly arms fall • Normal 'double slap' of hands against legs	Parkinsonism
Relax while clinician moves wrists and elbow joints slowly—ask patient to move head from side to side while assessing tone	• Degree of rigidity • Presence of 'cog-wheeling'	Parkinsonism
Hold arms out in front of them, close eyes and count backwards from 100	• Tremor • Any dystonic movements	• Tremor • Dystonias
With arms outstretched move fingers as though playing the piano	Rapidity and ease of movement	Parkinsonism
Look at observer, open mouth, then protrude tongue	Oro facial, bucco-lingual or other abnormal movements	Tardive dyskinesia
Stand still; if restless, ask whether 'in legs' (akathisia) or 'in head' (anxiety)	Restless, inability to stand still	Akathisia

treatment. Most commonly it affects the head and neck (torticollis) or produces spasm of the tongue, eyes, or back (opisthotonos). The *management* is anticholinergic medication, given intramuscularly or even intravenously if needed, and recovery is usually rapid. However, acute dystonia may, not unreasonably, result in an aversion to taking antipsychotic medication in the future.

In the era of typical antipsychotics, *akathisia*, a subjective and objective restlessness, was estimated to occur in about a quarter of people prescribed those medications. It is less common latterly, although it is seen with some newer antipsychotics, notably the dopamine partial agonist aripiprazole (it appears less troublesome with the newer partial agonist, brexpiprazole). Akathisia occurs reasonably early in treatment, and can be associated with distress or an increase in suicidal thinking. Patients describe it as 'an itch in the bone itself' and feel the impulse to move; it can interfere with sleep. *Management* includes reducing the dose of the offending medication, if appropriate. Benzodiazepines, beta-blockers, clonidine, or mirtazapine may be beneficial in the shorter term but if these fail, consideration should be given to a change of antipsychotic.

Parkinsonism occurs in up to a quarter of people on typical antipsychotics, and consists of the triad of bradykinesia, resting or 'pill rolling' tremor, and rigidity. Onset can be delayed by months after starting treatment. It is most common in women and the elderly, and where there is pre-existing damage to the brain. *Management* should follow a stepped approach. A dose reduction may help, treating at the minimum effective dose. It may also help to change to a second-generation antipsychotic. Anticholinergics will reduce the symptoms, but their longer-term use may add to the risk of developing tardive dyskinesia.

The most difficult antipsychotic-related movement disorder to manage is *tardive dyskinesia*. Classically this appears as a choreiform movement with tongue protrusion, although it can affect any muscle group. It often does not become evident for some years after starting medication and appears to be much less common with atypical antipsychotics, and especially with clozapine. The risk of tardive dyskinesia is relative to the degree of exposure to antipsychotics and seemingly increased by 'drug holidays'. Poor dentition can worsen it. Tardive dyskinesia is believed to be due to up-regulation of postsynaptic nigrostriatal dopaminergic receptors. *Management* is not easy. Because of the super-sensitivity, reducing antipsychotic dosage can temporarily exacerbate the problem. Clozapine can be used for difficult cases, although not everybody responds. There is a modest evidence base for tetrabenazine, benzodiazepines and vitamin E, which may be worth considering if other approaches are not successful, while valbenazine, which reduces the availability of dopamine in the synaptic cleft, has recently been approved by the US Food and Drug Administration for use in tardive dyskinesia.

What about cardiac risk?

As outlined in Chapters 2 and 3, people with schizophrenia are at high risk of premature mortality, and this is largely attributable to cardiovascular risk. While longer-term use of antipsychotics elevates such risks, antipsychotics can also pose shorter-term risks to cardiac health. Thus, people with psychotic illnesses taking antipsychotics are three times more likely to experience sudden cardiac death than the general population, the risk increasing with dose (Ray et al., 2009). Antipsychotics can alter cardiac contractility; we get a proxy measure of this using the QT interval on the electrocardiogram (ECG) tracing. This is a marker of cardiac repolarization, and if the QT interval (corrected for pulse rate) is high (≥450 msec for men, or 470 msec for women), then we infer an increased risk of cardiac arrhythmias or arrest. Different antipsychotics have various effects on the QTc interval, as shown in Fig. 6.2. An ECG is recommended on starting antipsychotics (Galletly et al., 2017) and if combining or using high-dose medications. Certain

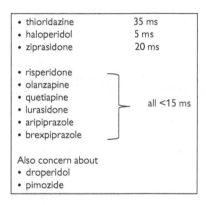

• thioridazine	35 ms
• haloperidol	5 ms
• ziprasidone	20 ms
• risperidone	
• olanzapine	
• quetiapine	
• lurasidone	all <15 ms
• aripiprazole	
• brexpiprazole	
Also concern about	
• droperidol	
• pimozide	

Fig. 6.2 Relative QTc prolongation of a range of antipsychotic medications

medications (e.g. ziprasidone) should be used with caution or avoided altogether in people with a long baseline ECG.

A more pervasive problem is long-term cardiovascular risk. This is affected by many factors, including the wider determinants of health, such as poverty and urban living, and exacerbated by lifestyle choices such as diet and sedentary behaviours (see Chapter 2). However, antipsychotic medications can have an additive contribution. In general, cardiometabolic effects such as weight gain and glucose and lipid dysregulation are more prominent with atypical and low-potency typical antipsychotics. Most people gain weight when starting an antipsychotic, but there is some variation between drugs in how quickly and to what extent this occurs, with drugs such as clozapine and olanzapine causing weight gain quite quickly. Box 6.1 shows relative 'ranking' of the antipsychotics in terms of propensity to weight gain.

Triglyceride levels can increase very rapidly with the introduction of certain antipsychotics, notably olanzapine and clozapine. Table 6.1 shows the relative propensity of the newer antipsychotics to hyperlipidaemia; of the more recently marketed agents, aripiprazole, brexpiprazole, and lurasidone all appear fairly benign in this regard. The increases are not simply correlated with weight gain and require specific monitoring and intervention, as shown in Box 6.1 (see Meyer (2013) for more information).

Given these data, it is clear that prevention of weight gain as well as recognition and rapid intervention for emergent cardiometabolic risk parameters is key from the very early stages of illness. Part of this is ensuring, from initiation, that the patient is informed about the rationale, efficacy, and likely side effects of any prescribed medication. The Appendix of this book provides detailed patient information material and espouses a 'shared decision-making' approach. By the time people are in their middle years with established

---

Box 6.1 Lipid abnormalities and antipsychotics

- ↑ TG and ↓ HDL associated with:
  - o Phenothiazines.
  - o Dibenzodiazepines (clozapine, olanzapine, quetiapine).
- ↑ TG rapid (e.g. 12% ↑ LDL after 6 weeks of olanzapine) and peaks around 1 year.
- ↑ TG not consistently associated with ↑ weight.

Clinical recommendations:

- Screening for risk factors (e.g. smoking, family history of cardiovascular disease, blood pressure, and weight).
- Baseline lipid profile and annually thereafter.
- With higher-risk antipsychotics, quarterly fasting TG and TC over first year.
- Advice about diet, lifestyle.
- If persistently high LDL, TG, TC—use statin.

HDL, high density lipoprotein; LDL, low density lipoprotein; TC, total cholesterol; TG, triglycerides

---

psychosis, half are obese, while three-quarters of men and 95% of women have central obesity, with high rates of dyslipidaemias (Gardner-Sood et al., 2015). Monitoring and treatment approaches to cardiometabolic risk are discussed in Chapters 7 and 8.

Is diabetes a side effect of antipsychotics?

An elevated risk of diabetes has been shown repeatedly among people with schizophrenia. Interestingly, such reports antedate the advent of antipsychotics and, as detailed in Chapter 2, might be indicative of an underlying vulnerability linked to schizophrenia itself. A recent meta-analysis (Pillinger et al., 2017) showed that at first presentation with psychosis, even before antipsychotics were prescribed, people with psychosis had higher fasting blood glucose and insulin levels as well as higher glucose in response to an oral glucose tolerance test, than matched controls.

However, it is clear that antipsychotics have an additive effect and that some agents are more strongly implicated than others (see Chapter 3 and Box 6.1). Underscoring this, Vancampfort et al. (2016) reported type 2 diabetes to be highly elevated in people with a severe mental illness with rates of 11.3% (95% confidence interval, 10.0–12.6%), while in antipsychotic-naïve patients, the prevalence was 2.9% (Vancampfort et al., 2016). The extent of worsening risk of diabetes in people with established schizophrenia was shown starkly in the study of Henderson et al. (2000) where, over a 5-year period, nearly a third of people on clozapine manifested diabetes.

It is therefore important to work with patients to understand this and to try to reduce the risk, for example, through promotion of healthy eating and regular exercise as part of their daily routine (see the Appendix of this book). Regular monitoring is imperative, expressly in individuals at heightened risk of diabetes, such as people who are already overweight (abdominal obesity being particularly concerning in this regard) and certain ethnic groups, such as people from the Indian subcontinent. Emerging evidence supports the use of metformin to both ameliorate weight gain as well as reduce insulin sensitivity in conjunction with 'high-risk' diabetogenic agents such as olanzapine and clozapine (see Chapters 3 and 8). Should diabetes evolve, a careful discussion needs to be had regarding whether a more 'metabolically friendly' antipsychotic can be used. Involvement of an endocrinologist and diabetes educator as well as the patient's general practitioner should all be part of the management strategy (see also Appendix).

What about prolactin?

Dopamine is otherwise known as prolactin inhibitory factor and blocking dopamine D2 receptors in the tuberoinfundibular tract in the brain (Fig. 6.1) increases circulating levels of prolactin. Interestingly, high levels of prolactin are also sometimes found in drug naïve first-episode patients, but less commonly so. The immediate effects of high prolactin are low libido, amenorrhoea, and galactorrhoea, with longer-term concerns about development of osteoporosis. There have also been suggestions that the risk of breast cancer is increased, but findings have been equivocal in this regard. Prolactin levels on antipsychotics are typically dose dependent, and there is considerable variation between individual drugs as to whether they will affect prolactin levels, largely related to the effect on the D2 receptor (see Box 6.1). Thus, amisulpride, risperidone, and paliperidone have the greatest effect, with aripiprazole, quetiapine, lurasidone, and clozapine having much less.

Many modern monitoring guidelines for people on antipsychotic agents suggest procuring a baseline (reference) prolactin level before commencing any medication, and then at least annual follow-up levels; some guidelines see this as necessary only for those antipsychotics which are relatively likely to elevate prolactin levels. It can be tricky to interpret prolactin levels as they vary between individuals as well as over time, notably in menstruating women. Thus, a careful and sensitively taken history of any prolactin-associated effects such as sexual dysfunction, menstrual irregularity, and breast engorgement and galactorrhoea, is also required.

Inder and Castle (2011) have suggested a staged approach to responding to raised prolactin levels in people with psychotic disorders. This is summarized in Box 6.2 (see Inder and Castle (2011) for more information). It is sensible, of course, to involve an endocrinologist in discussions about management.

> **Box 6.2** A staged approach to raised prolactin levels in people on antipsychotic agents
>
> • Engage endocrinologist and perform requisite tests, including pituitary fossa neuro-imaging, if indicated.
> • If clinically acceptable, lower dose or cease antipsychotic; reassess prolactin level as it should return to normal within days if due to the antipsychotic.
> • Consider switch to a 'prolactin-sparing' antipsychotic.
> • If cannot switch, consider addition of dopamine partial agonist aripiprazole.
> • Consider sex steroid replacement, with usual caveats and in consultation with endocrinologist.
> • Consider dopamine agonist (bromocriptine, cabergoline) with careful warning and monitoring regarding potential for exacerbation of psychosis.

Can sex be a problem?

Sexual problems are common in people with schizophrenia, as detailed in Chapter 4. Antipsychotic medication can be a contributory factor, with sexual dysfunction reported by about 50% of both men and women prescribed them (in part related to prolactin elevation: see 'What about prolactin?' section). It is also, however, seen in the first episode of psychosis and indeed in the drug-naïve prodrome (Marques et al., 2012).

Indeed, one of the best predictors of whether or not somebody reports sexual dysfunction is whether or not the clinician asks about it. Areas of enquiry are shown in Fig. 4.2 and Table 4.2. Sensitivity is required in this regard and it is important to establish the temporal sequence between the onset of the sexual problem and the commencement of the particular antipsychotic. It is also important to record which other medication the patient is on, as they might also have an impact: for example, many antidepressants reduce libido and delay orgasm. Furthermore, people with schizophrenia are at elevated risk of a number of medical conditions—vascular disease and diabetes are obvious ones—that can contribute to sexual problems. Alcohol abuse can also exacerbate sexual problems. Thus, taking a careful history and performing necessary tests should be part of a comprehensive appraisal and workup.

Involvement of the patient's sexual partner is also helpful in establishing relevant issues in the relationship that might be impacting sexual activity. Sexual dysfunction has a major effect on quality of life and can adversely affect relationships. It is thus important to take it seriously and address it. Strategies might include lifestyle advice, dose reduction or change of medication, and considering the use of a phosphodiesterase inhibitor. Involvement of relevant specialist colleagues should also be considered if simple strategies do not have benefit.

When is sedation a problem?

The antipsychotics were originally known as major tranquilizers. Older drugs, such as chlorpromazine, are highly sedative with marked antihistaminergic effects. This may be considered useful during the very acute phase of illness, but poses practical problems when trying to resume day-to-day activities. Clozapine and olanzapine are the most antihistaminergic of the second-generation antipsychotics, and therefore most inclined towards sedation. Quetiapine has weaker absolute binding to the histamine receptors, but its relative activity is greater for histamine than for the other receptors, and as a result it is highly sedating even at very low doses, with no major increase in sedation as the dose increases. Aripiprazole, on the other hand, has a low affinity for histaminergic receptors, and is not usually sedating—and in fact is activating in some people. If somebody is experiencing sedation, reducing the dose of medication often helps, but if this is not possible, then giving the greater dose at night or changing to a different preparation can be useful.

A related and often overlooked problem among people with schizophrenia is sleep apnoea. This is associated with diurnal fatigue as well as increased cardiovascular risk and requires specialist investigation (i.e. polysomnography) and advice about treatment (e.g. continuous positive airways pressure). For a fuller discussion, see Chapter 4.

What makes the approach to clozapine side effects special?

Clozapine is the only medication with a clear evidence base for the management of treatment-resistant schizophrenia. Therefore, if somebody needs clozapine, it is important to manage side effects, because they can be disabling and some can even prove fatal. The Appendix provides detailed information for patients commencing clozapine, while Fig. 6.3 reproduces a simple monitoring sheet for people starting clozapine.

The best known potentially dangerous side effect of clozapine is *agranulocytosis*. In the US, the latest clozapine guidance from the Food and Drug Administration is that treatment is interrupted if there is a suspected clozapine-induced neutropenia with an absolute neutrophil count less than 1000 cells/microlitre (<500 cells/ microlitre for those with benign ethnic neutropenia). The cut-off levels are higher in many other countries and local licensing conditions should be consulted when prescribing clozapine. Patients should generally not be re-challenged with clozapine if they have a clozapine-induced absolute neutrophil count less than 500 as recurrence is very likely. Drugs such as lithium and granulocyte colony-stimulating factor can increase the baseline white cell count, thus allowing people to remain within the monitoring range, but they will not prevent a true clozapine agranulocytosis.

Clozapine has other side effects that do not affect licensing. In the first few weeks there can be variations in blood pressure and tachycardia is ubiquitous. *Tachycardia* is usually benign and may be self-limiting although some patients find it drives anxiety symptoms. If benign but persistent it may need treatment (e.g. with

Fig. 6.3 Clozapine monitoring form.

Courtesy of St Vincent's Mental Health Service, Melbourne © David Castle.

ST. VINCENT'S MENTAL HEALTH
CLOZAPINE INITIATION
Form 1 of 2
Version: March 2012

ATTACH LABEL OR RECORD PATIENT DETAILS

SVH UR N°:

RAPID N°:

NAME:

SEX ☐ MALE ☐ FEMALE

DATE OF BIRTH:

INSTRUCTIONS: Complete for the first 18 weeks and then use the Metabolic Monitoring form on an ongoing basis. An authorised signed entry to be completed in the medical record progress notes for each measure on each occasion. Scan a copy after each entry, maintain original on site. When complete send original for scanning.

Clozapine Patient No. (CPN):

Patient Height: _____ (m)

Day (Insert Date of Procedure in unshaded cells)

Base Date		BASE	1	3	5	7	9	11	13	14	15	17	19	21	23	25	27	28	35	42
Key Investigations	FBE - Taken in the last 7 days / Monthly after 18 weeks — WCC																			
	Neutrophil																			
	Eosinophil																			
	Blood Group																			
	BHCG (Females where appropriate)																			
	LFTs																			
	U & Es																			
	Troponin I & T																	*		
	CRP																	*		
Metabolic Syndrome X	Fasting Blood Glucose																			
	Lipids (Cholesterol, LDL, HDL, TG)																			
	Weight (Kg)																			
	BMI = weight in kg by height in m²																			
	Waist Measurement (cm)																			
Cardiac	Echocardiogram (pre-commencement and as indicated*)																	*		
	ECG (pre-commencement and as indicated*)																			
Physical Observations	Temperature																			
	Blood Pressure																			
	Pulse																			
	Respiratory Rate																			
	Serum Clozapine																			

* If result normal report annually. If abnormal refer to Clozapine Policy

ST. VINCENT'S MENTAL HEALTH
CLOZAPINE INITIATION
Form 2 of 2
Version: March 2012

INSTRUCTIONS: Complete for the first 18 weeks and then use the Metabolic Monitoring Form on an ongoing basis.
An authorised signed entry to be completed in the medical record/progress notes for each measure on each occasion.
Scan a copy after each entry, maintain original on site.
When complete send original for scanning.

ATTACH LABEL OR RECORD PATIENT DETAILS

SVH UR N°:

SEX ☐ MALE ☐ FEMALE

NAME:

DATE OF BIRTH:

Clozapine Patient No. (CPN): _____ Patient Height: _____ (m) RAPID N°: _____

(Insert Dates of Procedure in unshaded cells)

		Week											
		7	8	9	10	11	12	13	14	15	16	17	18
Key Investigations	FBE - Taken in the last 7 days / Monthly after 18 weeks — WCC, Neutrophil, Eosinophil												
	Blood Group												
	BHCG (Females where appropriate)												
	LFTs												
	U&Es												
	Troponin I & T												
	CRP												
Metabolic Syndrome X	Fasting Blood Glucose												
	Lipids (Cholesterol, LDL, HDL, TG)												
	Weight (Kg)												
	BMI = weight in kg by height in m^2												
	Waist Measurement (cm)												
Cardiac	Echocardiogram (pre-commencement and as indicated*)					*							
	ECG (pre-commencement and as indicated*)												
Physical Observations	Temperature												
	Blood pressure												
	Pulse												
	Respiratory Rate												
	Serum Clozapine												

*An echocardiogram should only be done if clinically indicated – refer to Clozapine Policy

Fig. 6.3 Continued

a beta-blocker or ivabradine), as untreated persistent tachycardia may predispose to cardiomyopathy (Lally et al., 2014). If tachycardia occurs in conjunction with any symptoms such as fever, hypotension, chest pain, or a raised respiratory rate, an urgent cardiologist referral and investigation is needed, because of the possibility of myocarditis.

Myocarditis in association with clozapine occurs in 0.2–1.2% of patients, usually within the first few weeks. It is an immune-mediated idiosyncratic response and is associated with tachycardia, fever, autonomic instability, and shortness of breath. Confirmation of diagnosis includes transthoracic ultrasound or magnetic resonance imaging (see Kritharides et al., 2017). It can prove fatal and requires expert cardiologist care.

Cardiomyopathy is a rather more indolent problem with an incidence of about 5 per 10,000 patient years (Kritharides et al., 2017). Patients experience increasing fatigue and limitation of exercise capacity. Management may involve halting the clozapine but if this is clinically not feasible, regular echocardiographic monitoring and close liaison with a cardiologist is required.

Weight gain is often a substantial problem with clozapine. As well as lifestyle interventions, here has been some evidence to show that the addition of metformin or aripiprazole may be helpful (see Chapter 8).

Hypersalivation is common, especially at night resulting in a 'wet pillow': hyoscine is commonly used, as is pirenzepine, while a more recent trial suggests the use of metoclopramide (Kreinin et al., 2016).

Constipation is an interesting and under-recognized problem with many medications with powerful antimuscarinic properties, and perhaps most dramatically with clozapine (Shirazi et al., 2016). It is a highly uncomfortable problem for the patient and can be fatal. Yet clinicians often fail to ask about it proactively. It is important to encourage a high-fibre diet and to use laxatives (see Appendix), moving early to motility agents, as hypomotility is the core underlying problem.

Diurnal sedation, as outlined earlier, can be managed by changing the dose so the larger dose is at night-time; augmenting with aripiprazole may help. However, if one is given a larger dose at night-time, there may be a greater chance of developing enuresis, a common problem with many antipsychotics, but particularly with clozapine. *Enuresis* may respond to behavioural treatments or to desmopressin.

Doses of clozapine above 600 mg a day (or levels >500–600 micrograms /L) reduce the *seizure threshold*, so prophylactic anticonvulsant drugs are indicated. In practice, lamotrigine or valproate are commonly used. Valproate, however, can exacerbate weight gain and sedation and also increases the risk of neutropenia so should be used judiciously. It is also highly teratogenic so is best avoided in women of childbearing age.

So are antipsychotics bad for you?

With all the data outlined in this chapter about side effects of antipsychotics, one could wonder whether it would be better not to take them at all. However, apart from the obvious benefits in terms of mental health, people with schizophrenia also live longer when prescribed antipsychotics.

Two studies by Tiihonen et al. (2009, 2016) are particularly impressive, given their scale. They examine the whole populations of Finland and Sweden respectively. These authors confirmed that people with schizophrenia die younger than the general population. However, they also found that those individuals with schizophrenia who were taking antipsychotics lived longer than those not taking antipsychotics, while people on clozapine lived longest of all. In their later study, they reported that moderate- and high-dose antipsychotic and antidepressant exposure appeared to be protective, reducing overall mortality by 15–40%. Prescription of benzodiazepines, however, increased the mortality risk, highlighting the need for further research into whether that finding is a direct result of using benzodiazepines in schizophrenia, or is because of the known amplification in cardiovascular risk with anxiety. However, it appears that antipsychotics prescribed carefully and monitored closely and in collaboration with the patient should form part of a mortality reduction plan.

Conclusion

Antipsychotic medications are a key component of the treatment of schizophrenia and are often required long term. Individuals prescribed these medications often experience side effects and the management of these side effects is vital for quality of life. This is the epitome of personalized medicine, given the variation in side effects between drug classes, between individual drugs, and between patients. Prescribing requires thought and care; listening to feedback from patient and carers, and adjusting accordingly, sometimes repeatedly, in part of the recovery paradigm; and is reflected in shared decision-making processes (see Appendix).

REFERENCES

Galletly C, Castle DJ, Dark F, Humberstone V, Jablensky A, Killackey E, et al. (2016). Clinical practice guideline for the management of schizophrenia and related disorders. *Australian and New Zealand Journal of Psychiatry* 50, 410–472.

Gardner-Sood P, Lally J, Smith S, Atakan Z, Ismail K, Greenwood KE, et al. (2015). Cardiovascular risk factors and metabolic syndrome in people with established psychotic illnesses: baseline data from the IMPaCT randomized controlled trial. *Psychological Medicine* 45, 2619–2629.

Henderson DC, Cagliero E, Gray C, Nasrallah RA, Hayden DL, Schoenfeld DA, Goff DC (2000). Clozapine, diabetes mellitus, weight gain, and lipid abnormalities: a five-year naturalistic study. *American Journal of Psychiatry* 157, 975–981.

Inder WJ, Castle DJ (2011). Antipsychotic-induced hyperprolactinaemia. *Australian and New Zealand Journal of Psychiatry* 45, 830–837.

Jones PB, Barnes TRE, Davies L, Dunn G, Lloyd H, Hayhurst KP, et al. (2006). Randomized controlled trial of the effect on quality of life of second- vs first-generation antipsychotic drugs in schizophrenia: Cost Utility of the Latest Antipsychotic Drugs in Schizophrenia Study (CUtLASS 1). *Archives of General Psychiatry* 63, 1079–1087.

Kreinin A, Miodownik C, Mirkin V, Gaiduk Y, Yankovsky Y, Bersudsky Y, et al. (2016). Double-blind, randomized, placebo-controlled trial of metoclopramide for hypersalivation associated with clozapine. *Journal of Clinical Psychopharmacology* 36, 200–205.

Kritharides L, Chow V, Lambert TJR (2017). Cardiovascular disease in people with schizophrenia. *Medical Journal of Australia* 206, 91–95.

Lally J, Brook J, Dixon T, Gaughran F, Shergill S, Melikian N, MacCabe JH (2014). Ivabradine, a novel treatment for clozapine-induced sinus tachycardia: a case series. *Therapeutic Advances in Psychopharmacology* 4, 117–122.

Lally J, Gaughran F, Timms P, Curran SR (2016). Treatment-resistant schizophrenia: current insights on the pharmacogenomics of antipsychotics. *Pharmgenomics and Personalised Medicine* 9, 117–129.

Leucht S, Cipriani A, Spineli L, Mavridis D, Orey D, Richter F, et al. (2013). Comparative efficacy and tolerability of 15 antipsychotic drugs in schizophrenia: a multiple-treatments meta-analysis. *Lancet* 382, 951–962.

Lieberman JA, Stroup S, McEvoy J, Swartz MS, Rosenheck RA, Perkins DO, et al. (2005). Effectiveness of antipsychotic drugs in patients with chronic schizophrenia. *New England Journal of Medicine* 353, 1209–1223.

Marques TR, Smith L, Bonaccorso S, Gaughran F, Kolliakou A, Dazzan P, et al. (2012). Sexual dysfunction in people with prodromal signs of psychosis and in the first psychotic episode. *British Journal of Psychiatry* 201, 131–136.

Meyer JM (2013). Cardiovascular illness and hyperlipidaemia in patients with schizophrenia. In: Meyer JM, Nasrallah HA (eds) *Medical Illness in Schizophrenia*, pp. 53–80. Washington DC: American Psychiatric Publishing.

Pillinger T, Beck K, Gobjila C, Donocik JG, Jauhar S, Howes OD (2017). Impaired glucose homeostasis in first-episode schizophrenia: a systematic review and meta-analysis. *JAMA Psychiatry* 74(3), 261–269.

Ray WA, Chung CP, Murray KT, Hall K, Stein CM (2009). Atypical antipsychotic drugs and the risk of sudden cardiac death. *New England Journal of Medicine* 360, 225–235.

Shirazi A, Stubbs B, Gomez L, Moore S, Gaughran F, Flanagan RJ, et al. (2016). Prevalence and predictors of clozapine-associated constipation: a systematic review and meta-analysis. *International Journal of Molecular Science* 2, 17.

Tiihonen J, Lönnqvist J, Wahlbeck K, Klaukka T, Niskanen L, Tanskanen A, Haukka J (2009). 11-year follow-up of mortality in patients with schizophrenia: a population-based cohort study (FIN11 study). *Lancet* 2009, 620–27.

Tiihonen J, Mittendorfer-Rutz E, Torniainen M, Alexanderson K, Tanskanen A (2016). Mortality and cumulative exposure to antipsychotics, antidepressants, and benzodiazepines in patients with schizophrenia: an observational follow-up study. *American Journal of Psychiatry* 173, 600–606.

Vancampfort D, Correll CU, Galling B, Probst M, De Hert M, Ward PB, et al. (2016). Diabetes mellitus in people with schizophrenia, bipolar disorder and major depressive disorder: a systematic review and large scale meta-analysis. *World Psychiatry* 15, 166–174.

CHAPTER 7

A comprehensive monitoring approach to physical healthcare in people with schizophrenia

---

KEY POINTS

- There are numerous barriers to effective screening for and ongoing monitoring of physical health problems in people with schizophrenia.
- Monitoring of metabolic parameters should be seen as an imperative for mental health services and should be performed in conjunction with the patient and their general practitioner.
- Processes for communication between healthcare providers and processes to respond to abnormal physical health parameters should be agreed by all parties.

As has been outlined elsewhere in this book, there are numerous barriers to ensuring optimal physical healthcare for people with schizophrenia. We need to understand these barriers and work to overcome them. An initial step is to put in place strategies for effective screening for and ongoing monitoring of risk factors and early manifestations of physical health problems.

What are the barriers to monitoring and treating physical health problems in people with schizophrenia?

Barriers exist at the systems level, the clinician level, and the patient level (see Box 7.1).

Systems level

Despite so-called mainstreaming being a mantra for deinstitutionalized care and co-location of mental health and general hospitals being embraced widely across the world, there remains significant stigma which precludes people with schizophrenia receiving the same level of healthcare as people without a mental illness. For example, a study in the US showed that people with schizophrenia who had suffered an acute myocardial infarct were only 41% as likely as people without a mental illness to undergo cardiac catheterization (Druss

Box 7.1 Barriers to monitoring and treatment of physical health problems in people with schizophrenia

Systems level

- Stigma and lack of integration of services.
- Logistic issues related to blood collection and sharing of information.
- Lack of facilities within mental health services for physical health examinations and blood taking.
- Mental health services being separate from mainstream services.
- Emergency departments focusing on acute issues rather than longer-term secondary prevention.
- General practice being time-poor and focused on psychiatric rather than physical issues.
- Private practice being expensive and out of reach of many people with schizophrenia.

Clinician level

- Lack of clarity about role and 'whose job it is'.
- Therapeutic nihilism.
- Lack of knowledge and skills as to what should be assessed and how results should be acted upon.

Patient level

- Psychotic symptoms impairing organizational ability to participate in testing.
- Inability to articulate symptoms and to disentangle from psychotic symptoms.
- Logistic barriers due to lifestyle.
- Non-adherence.
- Cost.

Data from: *BMC Psychiatry*, 14, 2014, McKenna B, Furness T, Wallace E et al, 'The effectiveness of specialist roles in mental health metabolic monitoring: a retrospective cross-sectional comparative study, p. 234; *Australasian Psychiatry*, 18, 2010, Organ B, Nicholson E, DJ Castle, 'Implementing a physical health strategy in a mental health service, pp.456–459.

et al., 2000). The literature is replete with other examples of this kind (see Chapters 1 and 2).

Emergency departments tend to triage mental health down the acuity level such that people with mental illness wait for long periods before seeing a doctor and many simply leave before being seen. There is also a tendency for the focus of emergency departments to see people with a history of mental illness as 'psychiatric' patients and physical health issues are often not addressed adequately; and if they are, the focus is on acute issues rather than longer-term treatment and secondary prevention.

In general practice settings, the system tends to be set such that consultations are brief and focused on a particular 'presenting complaint'. In people with schizophrenia, this often means that the consultation is mainly or exclusively related to positive psychotic symptoms and neurological side effects of antipsychotic medications. This can leave the physical health problems undertreated.

Mental health service settings are often poorly equipped for physical health assessments and investigations, with a lack of appropriate equipment and staff being unsure of what to monitor and how to respond to results (Organ et al., 2010).

In many jurisdictions, private health insurance is simply out of reach of most people with schizophrenia and this can be a further barrier to high-quality healthcare. Patients thus face long waiting lists for 'elective' procedures such as joint replacements.

Clinician level

A major problem for many mental health clinicians is simply an underappreciation of the extent and importance of physical health problems among their patients, and a lack of clarity of role in terms of 'who should be doing what'. This is compounded by low levels of knowledge regarding what needs to be done in terms of both monitoring and acting upon abnormal results as well as problems in accessing appropriate services (Organ et al., 2010; Burton et al., 2016).

Regrettably, there is also a degree of what can only be termed 'nihilism' among some clinicians, regarding certain patients, in that there is an assumption that physical health checks and preventative physical health strategies will simply not be followed through on. All too often clinicians are so busy with—and focused on—assessing mental health symptoms and associated risks and disabilities that there seems to be no time to address physical health matters.

Many mental health clinicians—including psychiatrists—acknowledge the importance of physical health problems among their patients but see it as 'someone else's job' to address these aspects of care. For example, in a review of 995 psychiatrists in Australia, Laugharne et al. (2016) found that while 80% acknowledged metabolic problems to be a major concern in their patients, over half had no established protocols in place for even basic monitoring (for example, only 7% routinely checked patients' waist circumference).

Patient level

Cognitive impairment, negative symptoms, and formal thought disorder can make it difficult for the patient to enunciate their specific concerns and advocate for themselves regarding comprehensive care (Meyer and Nasrallah, 2003; and see Chapter 2). Pary and Barton (1988), for example, in a prospective study, found that fully 24 of 28 patients with schizophrenia were not able to name any of their physical health problems after 2 years' follow-up.

There is an obverse danger that certain symptoms that might be manifestations of a physical health malady are interpreted by the clinician as due to the primary mental health problem or as side effects of medication. For example, fatigue is common with sedating antipsychotics but might also be due to anaemia, endocrine abnormalities, or a malignancy. Similarly, constipation is seen commonly with medications with antimuscarinic effects but can also be a sign of, for example, colon malignancies.

Another side of this is that some people with schizophrenia either don't discuss physical health issues with medical professionals while others are excessively concerned with somatic problems and present continually with physical health symptoms, some of which may have delusional attribution. The latter group are particularly difficult to manage as there is a fine line between appropriate investigations and reassurance on the one hand, and over-investigation and reinforcement of aberrant somatization on the other.

Regarding monitoring and preventative strategies, people with schizophrenia might be reluctant or simply unable to follow through on medical recommendations. Regular blood tests, especially if they are fasting, can be difficult for the patient to organize and might be less likely to be followed through with if there is an associated cost. Also, there are substantial motivational and other barriers to health lifestyle interventions, including smoking cessation, as outlined in Chapters 5 and 8 of this book.

How can we monitor physical health parameters in people with schizophrenia?

One of the main decisions that must be reached is who does the monitoring. Another is what is to be monitored. A third is how results are shared. And finally, there is the issue of how results are acted upon (see Box 7.2).

In terms of who is responsible for the monitoring, it is best to see this as 'everyone's job', including clinicians, case workers, general practitioners (GPs), and patients and their carers. Provision of information is vital and this needs to be tailored for the particular needs of the audience. Examples of patient-directed versus clinician-directed educational materials are shown in Fig. 7.1 and 7.2.

Box 7.2 The fundamentals of physical health monitoring in people with schizophrenia

- Who is responsible?
- What is to be monitored?
- How will results be shared?
- How will the results be acted upon?

Looking after physical health
when you have a mental illness

Looking after physical health is important for everyone, but it can be an extra challenge when you have a mental illness.

This may be related to the symptoms of the illness or the side-effects of medication It may be because of smoking, not getting enough exercise, or other lifestyle factors. Physical health problems can also get over looked when everyone's focus is on looking after your mental health.

Whatever the reasons, people affected by mental illness often have some of the following problems:
• Weight gain, especially round the midriff
• High blood pressure
• High cholesterol
• High blood glucose levels.

If you are affected by a number of these problems, they may lead to heart disease, diabetes or other illnesses.

Having a mental illness, then, it makes it all the more important you look after your physical health too. Here are some simple but effective things that you can do to look after yourself.

A healthy lifestyle

A healthy lifestyle means enjoying yourself without risking your health. It can also mean stopping or reducing as much as possible things that are not healthy (such as smoking or abusing other drugs).

Having healthy everyday habits is one of the most powerful things you can do to reduce the risks associated with these problems:
• eating and drink healthily
• sleeping well
• managing stress
• staying in touch with others
• being physically active in your daily life.

Health Checks

It's a good idea to have a general health check when you first see your GP or psychiatrist. It's also important to have a check-up when you start on a new medication. Regular health checks are important for all of us, to identify early signs of any problems, so they can be dealt with promptly.

In a health check, the doctor may:

• ask about your lifestyle (for example, about smoking or how much exercise you get)
• ask about your physical health history and that of your family members
• Ask you about any sexual difficulties, or changes relating to periods or breast-milk
• check your blood pressure
• conduct blood tests for fats, sugars, live function and kidney function
• measure your waist (under 90 cm for women and under 100 cm for men is considered healthier)
• measure your weight
• examine you for involuntary muscle movements

(for example, restlessness, tremors or stiffness)

• listen to your heart-rate.

See a dentist and optometrist periodically too, to check the health of your teeth and eyes.

Monitoring and follow up

Seeing the same doctor regularly is ideal (or at least a doctor at the same clinic). It allows the doctor to get to know you, and makes it easier to talk about things. After the first health check, ask your doctor to follow up regularly on your general physical health and any specific conditions or concerns you have. Monitoring of some measurements, such as weight and waist circumference is best done every three months. Try doing this yourself too.

Fig. 7.1 Patient information material regarding physical healthcare.

Courtesy of SANE Australia, in conjunction with St Vincent's Mental Health Service, Melbourne © David Castle.

Taking action

Talk to your doctor about the risks that are specific to your illness, its treatment or your lifestyle. Ask them to test for a broad range of symptoms. Remember, you are entitled to these health checks. If any physical health problems are found, talk with your doctor about the options for improving your health.

These may include:
• starting a specific treatment
• considering a change of medication
• discussing lifestyle changes, like diet or sleep
• referral to low cost supports or programs, like dieticians or quit smoking programs.

Changes need not be dramatic to be successful.
Removing or decreasing even one risk factor can make a big difference. By taking control of your life in this way, you can make a big difference to your long-term health, and feel better too.

Shared Care—sharing information.
Often there are a number of services involved in looking after your health (for example, a GP, psychiatrist or other health professional). It's important that these all understand what the others are doing – to avoid duplication of tests, for example, and that what they are doing is coordinated in your best interests.

Benefits of prevention and detection
• *Feeling better mentally*
Being physically healthy is good for your mental health.

• *Fewer health problem*
Lowering risk of developing illnesses

• *Getting help sooner*
Identifying problems early, so they can be treated sooner.

• *Taking control*
Getting regular health checks helps you feel you are taking control of your life.

Fig. 7.1 Continued

Fast facts
• Looking after physical health is even more important for people affected by mental illness.

• People affected by mental illness are often affected by health problems such as being overweigh or high blood pressure. There may also be a challenge with issues such as poor diet and lack of exercise.

• It's important to talk to your doctor about your physical as well as mental health.

• A healthy lifestyle can make a big difference to your mental as well as physical health – for example, improving diet, sleep habits and staying in touch with other people.

• Ask your doctor for a regular physical health check, including weight and waist measurements, blood pressure and blood tests.

• If any health problems are found, talk to your doctor about the best treatments, and also what you can do yourself to improve your health.

• Looking after your physical as well as mental health means you will feel better, are likely to have fewer health problems later in life, and will get help sooner for any which arise. It also helps you take control of your life, and improve your own health.

OVERVIEW
- people with severe mental illness are at increased risk for a number of medical conditions.
- these are often undetected and untreated, with subsequent elevated morbidity & mortality.
- Routine monitoring of weight, glucose and serum lipids are required.
- optimal medical care, and extra monitoring in high risk individuals, is required.

- Monitor weight, BMI, abdominal girth (and triglycerides, fasting glucose, blood pressure)
- Behavioural approach (Wirshing et al, 1999)
  - weight every visit (1–4 weeks)
  - diary of food intake & dietician advice
  - exercise classes
- Medications
  - select antipsychotic or switch to agent with less propensity to weight gain
  - Some potential weight-loss agents available. Refer for medical review.

Obesity

- **BMI (Body Mass Index)**
  = Weight in kg / height in m^2
- **BMI >30kg /m^2 = "obese"** (25–29 = "overweight")
- **Related to increased risk for:**
  - diabetes
  - hypertension
  - cardiovascular disease (CVD)
  - arthritis
  - breast cancer
- **Significant social stigma**

Obesity in Mental Illness

- **Rates > general population**
- **Driven by Diet & Lifestyle + Medications**
  - Antipsychotics
    - 10 week data (Alison et al, 1996)
    - Clozapine 4.4kg
    - Olanzapine 4.1kg
    - Risperidone 2.1kg
    - Ziprasidone 0.04kg
    - Aripiprazole –1.0kg over 26 week
    - Ziprasidone essentially weight neutral
      (Carsson et al, 2002)
    - possibly worse in adolescents
      (Theisen et al, 2001)
  - Valproate
  - Lithium
- **Significant reason for non-adherence to medication**

Management

- Warn patient & institute diet/exercise regime early

Hyperlipidaemia

Normal ranges:
- HDL/LDL <3.5
- Total cholesterol/HDL <4.5
- linear relationship between CVD and serum cholesterol (Stamler et al, 1986)
- reducing total cholesterol (TC) and low density lipoprotein (LDL) significantly reduces CVD risk
- use of statins effective (target 3-hydroxy 3-methylglutarylcoenzyme A—HMGCOA reductase involved in cholesterol synthesis)

Hyperlipidaemia & Antipsychotics

- ↑ TG and ↓ high density lipoprotein (HDL) associated with
  - phenothiazines
  - dibenzodiazepines (clozapine, olanzapine, quetiapine)
    (Meyer, 2003)
- ↑ TG rapid (eg. 12% ↑ LDL after 6 weeks of olanzapine) ... and peaks around 1 year (Glick et al, 2001)
- ↑ TG not consistently associated with ↑ weight

Clinical Recommendations

- screening for risk factors (eg. smoking, family history of CVD, bp and weight)
- baseline lipid profile and annually thereafter
- with higher-risk antipsychotics, quarterly fasting TG & TC over first year
- advice about diet, lifestyle
- if persistently high LDL, TG, TC, use statin
  (Meyer, 2003)

Fig. 7.2 Fact sheets for mental health staff outlining requirements and processes for physical health monitoring.
Courtesy of St Vincent's Mental Health Service, Melbourne © David Castle.

Glucose Intolerance & Diabetes

Normal range 4–7 mmol/L

<u>American Diabetic Association (ADA) Criteria:</u>

Clinical Factors
+ random glucose	≥ 11.1 mmol/l
or fasting glucose	≥ 7 mmol/l
or GTT glucose	≥ 11.1 mmol/l

For glucose intolerance
fasting glucose   >5 mmol/l

Type I diabetes = problem of insulin
secretion
Type II diabetes = insulin resistance
(hepatic, skeletal muscle, adispose tissue)
(Lebovitz, 2001)

Factors Associated with Type II Diabetes

■ genetic predisposition
(Lebovitz, 2001)

■ central obesity
■ excess caloric intake
■ high fat ingestion
■ ↓ physical activity

 PLUS: Medications, by

■ ↑ appetite
■ altered fat distribution
■ sedation - ↓ activity
■ interfere with insulin cascade
■ ↑ FFA (free fatty acid) release from
fatty tissue

Diabetes & Antipsychotics

Clozapine 5-year Study of
101 participants:
(Henderson et al, 2000)
■ Prior diabetes exacerbated 36 new
cases

Olanzapine

■ Case reports of diabetes & DKA (dia-
betic ketoacidosis)
■ Case reports of diabetes resolving once
Olanzapine stopped

Fig. 7.2 Continued

Risperidone

■ A few reports, mostly in people already
predisposed

Quetiapine

■ possible modest increase in risk (?relat-
ed to weight gain)

Aripiprazole

■ no evidence to suggest any elevated risk

Ziprasidone

■ no evidence to suggest increased risk

Screening & Monitoring
(Henderson et al, 2000)
■ risk assessment (family history, obesity, etc.)
■ baseline fasting glucose (and other bloods)
■ advice regarding diet and exercise

■ regular fasting glucose every 6 months
and more frequently if risk factors, eg.
   − age > 45yrs
   − ethnicity (Indian, African)
   − obese
   − Family history of diabetes
   − prior elevated plasma glucose
   − prior gestational diabetes
■ if patient develops diabetes
   − diet & exercise and general measures
   − consider change of antipsychotic to
lowrisk agent
   − treat & monitor

Hyperprolactinaemia

Normal range 0-20 ng/ml
Pregnant Women 10-300 ng/ml
■ notably with typicals and risperidone,
amisulpride
■ association with sexual dysfunction &
menstrual irregularities
■ galactorrhoea / breast enlargement
■ long term osteoporosis?
■ ? ↑ risk of breast cancer

Screening & Monitoring
□ Suggest baseline and annual prolactin
levels for prolactin-elevating antipsychotics
□ If markedly/persistently high − med-
ical/endocrine review; if any side
effects of concern consider switch to
other antipsychotic.

Cardiac

- Prolonged QTc due to effects on K+ channels delay repolarization

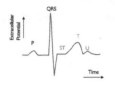

QTc and Antipsychotics
- Resting QTc typically: Females < 420 ms Males < 430 ms
- Risk of sudden death (torsades de pointes, ventricular fibrillation) at QTc > 500 ms

Which Antipsychotics Affect Cardiac Conduction?

Thioridazine	35 ms
Haloperidol	5 ms
Ziprasidone	20 ms
Risperidone	
Olanzapine	all < 15 ms
Quetiapine	

Also concern about
- Droperidol
- Pimozide

Screening & Monitoring
- Baseline and at least annual ECG for patients with any pre-existing cardiac problem and for all patients starting Ziprasidone.

Disclaimer
The information contained in this leaflet is not intended to be a substitute for medical care. Decisions regarding treatment are complex medical decisions requiring the independent, informed decision of an appropriate health care professional. Reference to any drug or substance does not imply recommendation by the authors who accept no responsibility for any clinical untoward event that may arise from following the recommendations contained herein.

This Fact Sheet has been prepared by Professor David Castle, Chair of Psychiatry, St. Vincent's Mental Health and The University of Melbourne; formatted by Malinda Edwards.

Fig. 7.2 Continued

What is required for monitoring?

At the bare minimum, tools required for monitoring encompass scales that can weigh over 100 kg, a blood pressure cuff that can accommodate a large upper arm circumference, and a tape measure for waist circumference. More sophisticated measurement materials could include scales that measure percentage body fat and calipers for skinfold thickness. Staff training in how to use these tools is crucial. Waist circumference is particularly susceptible to measurement error and a standardized procedure should be followed, as outlined in Box 7.3 (see Galletly et al. (2012) for further information).

Recording and sharing of information between health professionals and the patient is imperative if aberrant findings are to be effectively acted upon. A combination of paper and pencil and electronic records is usual and can lead to duplication and confusion if both are not kept up to date synergistically. In terms of patient empowerment, a copy of the results should be made available for their own records; this also allows them to share the information with health

> **Box 7.3** Measurement of waist circumference
>
> - Locate top of hip bone.
> - Place tape measure evenly around abdomen at level of hip bone.
> - Tape measure should be snug but not compressing the skin.
> - Ask patient to breathe out.
> - Take measure at end of normal expiration.

professionals with whom they have contact. Fig. 7.3 shows a simplified template that can be provided to the patient as their own record, as well as being a clinician tool.

While all these processes might seem routine and mundane, many mental health services do not follow them minutely. Continual staff upskilling and reminders to staff and patients is required. Poster displays in waiting areas and inclusion of physical health monitoring as part of clinical reviews can help reinforce these messages. These combined efforts can reap dividends. For example, serial audits in an Australian mental health service found that rates of adherence to measurements such as weight and blood glucose and lipids improved from under 10% to 54% and 63%, respectively, after a concerted educational campaign. Waist circumference measurement was, however, performed in only 7% of patients, despite each clinician in the service having been provided with a tape measure (Organ et al., 2010).

Much more impressive results were achieved in a service which employed a nurse specifically to oversee metabolic monitoring. In that context, metabolic monitoring rates of 78% were achieved and specific referral pathways were established for those patients found to be at high risk (McKenna et al., 2014). Those authors concluded that such designated specialist roles are required within mental health services to ensure high levels of metabolic monitoring as well as local tailored physical health interventions. Regrettably, funding agencies mostly do not see this as an imperative and such dedicated personnel are all too rare in clinical services.

How should results be acted upon?

The process of monitoring is useless in itself. The key is to ensure that any concerning results are appropriately acted upon. This is often the biggest area of neglect at a service level and requires concerted interagency collaboration. In many jurisdictions, the GP is the main locus of care for physical health issues and it is important to ensure patients with a mental illness have a regular GP and that tests results are shared with their GP. The GP can enact appropriate physical health treatments and monitor the efficacy thereof, or arrange on-referral to other specialists as required. An outline of physical health interventions is supplied in Chapter 8 of this book.

ST VINCENT'S MELBOURNE
METABOLIC MONITORING
MENTAL HEALTH

Instructions for Use:
This form should be used for all mental health patients.
More frequent monitoring may be required if there is a change in medication or as clinically indicated.
An authorised signed entry to be completed in the medical record progress notes for each measure on each occasion.

Scan when completed.

Surname: _____
Given Name: _____
D.O.B.: _____

INSERT RESULT IN EACH CELL		Base Date __/__/__	3 Months __/__/__	6 Months __/__/__	12 Months __/__/__	18 Months __/__/__	24 Months __/__/__	30 Months __/__/__	36 Months __/__/__
	Height (m)								
	Weight (in kg)								
	BMI = weight in kg by height in m².								
	Waist (cm)								
	Blood Pressure								
Physical & Metabolic	Fasting Blood Glucose								
	Lipids (Chol, LDL, HDL, TG)								
	LFT (ALP, GGT, ALT)								
(for all patients on psychotropic medications)	U&E (Na, K, eGFR, Ca, PO4)								
	FBE (Hb, WCC, Platelet, Neutrophil)								
	TFTs (TSH, T4, T3)								
	Prolactin								
	Vitamin D								
	Others (e.g.: BHCG, HbA1c, CRP, TroponinIT)								
Cardiac	ECG								
	Echocardiogram (if indicated)								
Main psychotropic medications	1.								
	2.								
	3.								
Medication levels	e.g.: Lithium, Clozapine								
	Interventions								
	Print name & signature of doctor completing this entry:								

METABOLIC MONITORING FORM - MENTAL HEALTH - ST VINCENT'S MELBOURNE

Fig. 7.3 Metabolic monitoring template.
Courtesy of St Vincent's Mental Health Service, Melbourne © David Castle.

Other individuals and services who should be included, as required, are dieticians, exercise physiologists, endocrinologists, and cardiologists. The scope of who needs to be involved depends upon the individual patient as well as local availability. It is also important that the patients themselves (and carers, where appropriate) are made aware of the results of investigations and of the actions they can take to effect healthier living. The Appendix of this book provides materials for use with patients and carers in this regard.

Conclusion

Monitoring of metabolic parameters should be seen as an imperative for mental health services and should be performed in conjunction with the patient and their GP. Processes for communication between healthcare providers and processes to respond to abnormal physical health parameters should be agreed by all parties.

REFERENCES

Burton A, Walters K, Atkins L, Howard M, Michie S, Peveler R, et al. (2016). Barriers, facilitators, and effective interventions for lowering cardiovascular disease risk in people with severe mental illness: evidence from a systematic review and focus group study. *Lancet* 388, S30.

Druss BG, Bradford DW, Rosenheck RA, Radford MJ, Krumholz HM (2000). Mental health disorders and use of cardiovascular procedures after myocardial infarction. *JAMA* 283, 506–511.

Galletly C, Foley D, Waterreus A, Watts G, Castle D, McGrath J, et al. (2012). Cardiometabolic risk factors in people with psychosis: the second Australian national survey of psychosis. *Australian and New Zealand Journal of Psychiatry* 46, 753–761.

Laugharne J, Waterreus A, Castle DJ, Dragovic M (2016). Screening for metabolic syndrome in Australia: a national survey of psychiatrists' attitudes and reported practice in patients prescribed antipsychotic drugs. *Australasian Psychiatry* 24, 62–66.

McKenna B, Furness T, Wallace E, Happell E, Stanton R, Platania-Phung C, et al. (2014). The effectiveness of specialist roles in mental health metabolic monitoring: a retrospective cross-sectional comparative study. *BMC Psychiatry* 14, 234.

Meyer JM, Nasrallah HA (2003). Issues surrounding medical care for individuals with schizophrenia: the challenge of dual neglect by patients and the system. In: Meyer JM, Nasrallah HA (eds) *Medical Illness and Schizophrenia*, pp. 1–12. Washington, DC: American Psychiatric Publishing, Inc.

Organ B, Nicholson E, Castle D (2010). Implementing a physical health strategy in a mental health service. *Australasian Psychiatry* 18, 456–459.

Pary RJ, Barton SN (1988). Communication difficulty of patients with schizophrenia and physical illness. *Southern Medical Journal* 81, 489–490.

CHAPTER 8

Interventions for metabolic problems in people with schizophrenia

> **KEY POINTS**
>
> - Weight gain and metabolic risk is common in people with schizophrenia.
> - An array of psychosocial interventions and various medication strategies can be effective in ameliorating risk.
> - Strategies that empower the patient to effect a more healthy lifestyle should be encouraged.
> - Choice of more 'metabolically friendly' antipsychotics should, where possible, be given precedence by clinicians.

It is clear that there are major unmet needs in terms of helping people with schizophrenia deal with their physical health problems. Chapter 7 of this book outlined how crucial it is for services to have concerted monitoring processes in place to ensure risk factors are picked up and assessed longitudinally. This chapter focuses on general physical health strategies to assist patients to lead as healthy a life as possible and provides a framework for more specific therapeutic interventions.

What frameworks enable physical health service delivery in people with schizophrenia?

Liu et al. (2017) have produced an overall approach to helping structure a holistic response to the physical health burden associated with schizophrenia. This is shown in Box 8.1. This chapter concentrates on the clinical service delivery component of this framework, but the broader issues raised by Liu and colleagues is important to contextualize any set of interventions.

There are a number of different clinical approaches to addressing physical health problems among people with schizophrenia. One set of mechanisms is encompassed under the term 'integrated self-management'. Whiteman et al. (2016) recently reviewed integrated self-management interventions for addressing physical health problems among people with serious mental illness. Fifteen studies were included (nine were randomized controlled trials (RCTs)), covering a range of strategies, including telehealth, peer programmes, life goal-setting,

---

Box 8.1 Framework for a response to physical health issues among the mentally ill

- Individual-focused interventions:
  - o Mental health disorder management
  - o Physical health treatment
  - o Lifestyle behavioural interventions.
- Health system-focused interventions:
  - o Service delivery (screening, care coordination, integrated delivery).
- Community level and policy-focused interventions:
  - o Social support
  - o Stigma reduction
  - o Policy-level interventions.

Data from *World Psychiatry*, 16, 2017, Liu NH, Daumit GL, Dua T et al, 'Excess mortality in persons with severe mental disorders: a multilevel intervention framework and priorities for clinical practice, policy and research agendas', pp. 30–40, The World Psychiatric Association.

---

and 'targeted training'. While most of these programmes were feasible to implement and showed acceptability, they generally did not produce clinically effective outcomes. Whiteman et al. (2016) identified costs, workforce issues, and requirement for long-term interventions to be substantial potential barriers to implementation. A more encouraging set of outcomes has been reported from programmes targeting nutrition (Teasdale et al., 2017).

The challenge, then, is to build on those elements of programmes that have proven effective, and to deliver them in a manner that educates and empowers patients. There is also a challenge to ensure that the various parts of what are often rather complex and dislocated systems, work together towards ensuring the specific and particular needs of each individual are achieved. Ongoing monitoring and support are required, as is communication between different healthcare providers.

Specific programmes

A specific self-management programme that seeks to help people address both mental and physical health through building a set of skills and supporting self-efficacy is the Optimal Health Program (OHP) (Ski et al., 2016). The programme can be delivered one-to-one or be group-based and follows a semi-structured format, as shown in Box 8.2.

One of the virtues of the OHP is that it has enough flexibility to enable the individual to prioritize areas of specific concern to them and also to understand the interactions between the physical and mental health aspects of their lives. It is a generic platform that has its genesis in the mental health arena but which explicitly deals with physical health problems as well. A specific aspect is the

Box 8.2 Overall structure of the Optimal Health Program modified for chronic disease

- Session 1. Understanding optimal health: six domains of health.
- Session 2. Implications of chronic disease: strengths and vulnerabilities.
- Session 3. Communication strategies: understanding and monitoring impact.
- Session 4. Pharmacology and metabolic monitoring: medication and health.
- Session 5. Community supports and strategies: identification of key health partnerships.
- Session 6. Change enhancement: establishing proactive avenues for change.
- Session 7. Integrated health plans: creative problem-solving and planning.
- Session 8. Advance care planning: maintaining well-being.
- Session 9. Booster session.

Data from *Trials*, 17, 2016, Ski CF, Thompson DR, Castle DJ, 'Trialling of an optimal health program (OHP) across chronic disease', p 447.

establishment of a network of support people (called 'collaborative partners') who include health practitioners and others and who work to support the individual and ensure a coherent communication plan is adhered to. Inclusion of peer workers is also possible, if the patient desires this.

A somewhat different approach is to build upon programmes established for people in the general population who have chronic diseases (e.g. diabetes), and adapt them for use in people with a mental illness. An example is the Chronic Disease Self-Management Program (CDSMP) (Lorig et al., 2001), a six-session intervention facilitated by peers and which emphasizes, inter alia, building self-confidence, action planning, and problem-solving. Druss et al. (2010) performed a RCT of a mental health adaptation of the CDSMP in 80 people with a broad range of mental illnesses and reported improvements associated with the CDSMP (relative to controls) in 'activation' and also in use of primary care; however, there were no demonstrable benefits in physical activity, medication adherence, or health-related quality of life.

In separate work, Goldberg et al. (2013) developed 'Living Well', again based on the CDSMP but with a focus on use more specifically in people with psychotic disorders. The programme was designed to be delivered by either two mental health peer workers or one peer worker and one mental health clinician and was extended to 13 weekly sessions. Box 8.3 shows an outline of the programme. Throughout, there is also an emphasis on how mental health and general medical services can be effectively negotiated in a coordinated manner.

Goldberg et al. (2013) performed a RCT of 'Living Well' in 63 people with a psychotic illness and at least one chronic medical illness (e.g. diabetes, asthma, chronic obstructive airways disease, or cardiovascular disease). Those randomized to the active intervention showed improvements relative to controls on measures of illness self-management, physical and emotional well-being, and

Box 8.3 Outline of the 'Living Well' programme

Sessions 1–3: self-management strategies

- Action planning
- Peer feedback and support
- Modelling
- Problem-solving.

Sessions 4–13: specific disease management strategies

- Nutrition
- Exercise
- Sleep
- The role of medication
- Dealing with addictive behaviours.

Data from *Psychiatric Services*, 64, 2013, Goldberg RW, Dickerson F, Lucksted A et al, 'Living Well: an intervention to improve self-management of medical illness for individuals with serious mental illness', pp. 51–57, American Psychiatric Association.

general health functioning. Self-efficacy also improved in the intervention group. Not all gains were sustained at 2-month post-intervention follow-up, leading the authors to suggest that booster sessions should be considered to enhance longer-term benefits. The inclusion of peer workers in this model is particularly interesting, given the increasing interest in peer worker involvement in mental health services in general.

A number of programmes have adopted a more targeted approach to cardio-vascular risk factors in particular. For example, Baker et al. (2009) developed a comprehensive 'Healthy Lifestyles' intervention for obese smokers with a serious mental illness (Box 8.4). In their pilot study of 43 patients, there were significant improvements in smoking, weight, exercise, and overall coronary health disease risk profile, but no change was noted in blood pressure or cholesterol levels. It should be noted that the antismoking mediation used in this trial was nicotine replacement therapy: other medication strategies for smoking cessation are outlined in Chapter 5.

Of interest is that in a large RCT (*n* = 235) building on this work, Baker et al. (2015) confirmed these overall findings but showed that a control group who received a predominantly telephone-based education and support programme did just as well on the outcomes of interest. This begs the question of what is a 'bare minimum' intervention that might cost-effectively help most people with schizophrenia reduce their cardiovascular risk? It also remains to be shown whether Internet-based interventions could meet the needs of a proportion of such patients. There are obvious advantages to Internet treatments including reach to rural and remote locations as well as cost. However, there is a degree of self-discipline involved in following these programmes and

---

Box 8.4 Synopsis of 'Healthy Lifestyles' intervention

- Session 1: motivational interviewing, decisional balance, goal setting, treatment planning, self-monitoring homework assignment.
- Session 2: activity planning, identification of 'high risk' situations, planning quite date, coping with urges, education about withdrawal symptoms, supply of NRT (nicotine replacement), homework.
- Session 3: reinforcement of quit attempt and behaviour change, coping with cravings, engagement of support person, education about healthy eating and shopping.
- Session 4: identify unhelpful thought and educate about cognitive restructuring.
- Session 5: relaxation, problem solving, education about take-away foods.
- Session 6: coping skills for psychotic symptoms, anger and frustration, assertiveness and cigarette and food refusal.
- Session 7: relapse prevention planning.
- Session 8: review relapse prevention plan as well as monitoring and reward achievement.

Reproduced from Baker A, Richmond R, Castle D, 'Coronary Heart Disease Risk Reduction Intervention Among Overweight Smokers with a Psychotic Disorder: Pilot Trial', *Australian and New Zealand Journal of Psychiatry*, 43, 2, pp. 129–135. Copyright (2009) SAGE Publications.

---

clinician (or peer) support as an adjunct could arguably enhance engagement and outcomes.

Medications: how should psychotropic choice respond to physical health risk?

One of the most important aspects of the care of people with a mental illness is, where feasible, to choose psychotropic agents that will not place them at excess extra risk of physical health problems. Chapter 6 of this book makes clear that antipsychotic agents in particular differ widely in terms of their propensity to cause weight gain, diabetes, and hyperlipidaemia on the one hand; and hyperprolactinaemia on the other. It is important to add that there are no accurate predictors of who will develop which of these effects on which agent. Indeed, a proportion of people on olanzapine and clozapine do not gain weight and remain at metabolic low risk even after prolonged exposure to such drugs. But they are the exceptions and clinicians should warn patients about the likely range of side effects associated with each medication and enter a shared decision-making process with the patient (as outlined in the Appendix of this book).

Also, given that antipsychotics are generally used over prolonged periods, treating in the short term with a view to the long term is a useful rubric. Hence, using olanzapine in a first-episode psychosis patient in the acute phase all too often leads to longer-term exposure to that agent, with concomitant metabolic risks. It might be better to start with a more metabolically 'friendly' antipsychotic (see Chapter 6) and use olanzapine only if others fail or are not tolerated (Correll et al., 2014; Galletly et al., 2016).

Clozapine is worthy of particular consideration in this context. It remains a uniquely effective agent for some people, but does carry risk in terms of neutropenia and the metabolic syndrome as well as rarer but sometimes fatal cardiac problems (myocarditis, cardiomyopathy). Hence, particular care needs to be taken to initiate this agent slowly and to monitor for side effects over the long term, as detailed in Chapter 6.

It is not just antipsychotics that can cause or exacerbate physical health problems in people with schizophrenia. For example, weight gain is a recognized side effect of the antidepressant mirtazapine, the anticonvulsant/mood stabilizer sodium valproate (divalproate), and lithium. Clinicians need to be aware of these issues and try to avoid combinations of medications that could cause accumulated risk.

What medications might help address physical health problems in people with schizophrenia?

Much of the early literature on medication interventions that might ameliorate physical health problems in people with schizophrenia relied on evidence from the non-psychiatric population. This has potential shortfalls in that some such medications might exacerbate psychiatric symptoms by interaction with psychotropics and/or through direct psychiatric effects. However, there is an emerging literature on medications that can help address (to some extent at least) weight gain and associated hyperlipidaemia and glucose intolerance and which are safe to use in conjunction with antipsychotics in people with schizophrenia. These are summarized in Table 8.1.

Of the options shown in Table 8.1, the use of metformin, a biguanide anti-hyperglycaemic agent approved for use in type 2 diabetes, has gained particular favour with many clinicians as it is well tolerated, cheap, and relatively safe. It also has an emerging evidence base in people with schizophrenia. For example, Jarskog et al. (2013) performed a RCT of metformin (titrated up to 1000 mg twice daily) in 148 clinically stable, overweight (body mass index (BMI) > 26) individuals with schizophrenia or schizoaffective disorder. Over 16 weeks of treatment, metformin was associated with 3 kg (95% CI, 2–4) weight loss (compared to 1 kg (0–2) in the placebo group) as well as improvements in triglyceride and haemoglobin A1c levels. Transient gastrointestinal upset was the most common side effect associated with metformin and most patients tolerated this. An issue raised by the trial authors is whether these benefits would continue to accrue over longer-term exposure to metformin; this requires research but clinical wisdom suggests ongoing use of the agent if it is well tolerated and beneficial in the shorter term. One caution is a small

Table 8.1 Potential medication strategies to ameliorate metabolic syndrome risk in schizophrenia

Medication	Comments
Metformin	Associated with modest weight loss and decreased insulin sensitivity; safe and few side effects
Phentermine	Relatively contraindicated in schizophrenia as risk of exacerbation of psychosis
Sibutramine	Modest efficacy for weight gain; potential for exacerbation of psychosis
Topiramate	Helpful for weight loss in some patients; can cause cognitive problems
Orlistat	Requires strict dietary adherence; no good evidence for efficacy in schizophrenia patients
Reboxetine	Useful for weight loss in some patients; risk of noradrenergic side effects
Lorcaserin	No published trials in schizophrenia
Naltrexone/bupropion combination	Still in development; no published trials in schizophrenia

Data from *American Journal of Psychiatry*, 170, 2013, Jarskog LF, Hamer RM, Catellier DJ et al, 'Metformin for weight loss and metabolic control in overweight outpatients with schizophrenia and schizoaffective disorder', pp. 1032–1040, American Psychiatric Association.

risk of lactic acidosis, expressly in the context of renal insufficiency, so renal function requires monitoring as well.

Another popular medication strategy is the addition of the dopamine partial agonist aripiprazole in patients who have responded well but gained weight on metabolically more problematic drugs (notably clozapine). In reviewing the literature on aripiprazole as an adjunct to other antipsychotics, Zheng et al. (2016) found 55 RCTs including 4457 patients. Aripiprazole was associated with improved psychopathology scores as well as a mean 5.08 kg (95% CI, 3.02–7.14) reduction in weight (9 RCTs; n = 505) and improvement in BMI of 1.78 (95% CI, 1.31–2.25) (14 RCTs; n = 809).

What other weight loss strategies are there?

A variety of surgical procedures are now commonplace in obesity management settings, but there are few reports of patients with schizophrenia undergoing such procedures. Hamoui et al. (2004) reported five morbidly obese individuals (mean BMI 54) with schizophrenia who underwent duodenal switch (n = 3), sleeve gastrectomy (n = 1), and biliopancreatic diversion (n = 1). The authors report favourable weight loss outcomes without adverse psychiatric effects. Clearly, surgical interventions for obesity need patients to be carefully worked up and educated about the procedure and the dietary requirements post procedure. Schizophrenia should not be an exclusion criterion per se but extra care should be taken, including close monitoring of mental state post procedure. Further studies over longer time periods are required to better understand the place of such procedures in this clinical context.

Conclusion

While weight gain and metabolic risk is common in people with schizophrenia, various strategies can be helpful in ameliorating risk. These include psychosocial interventions and various medication strategies. Choice of more 'metabolically friendly' antipsychotics should, where possible, be given precedence by clinicians.

REFERENCES

Baker A, Richmond R, Castle D, Kulkarni J, Kay-Lambkin F, Sakrouge R, et al. (2009). Coronary heart disease risk reduction intervention among overweight smokers with a psychotic disorder: pilot trial. *Australian and New Zealand Journal of Psychiatry* 43, 129–135.

Baker A, Richmond R, Kay-Lambkin FJ, Filia S, Castle D, Williams J, et al. (2015). Randomised controlled trial of a healthy lifestyle intervention among smokers with psychotic disorders. *Nicotine and Tobacco Research* 17, 946–954.

Correll CU, Robinson DG, Schooler NR, Brunette MF, Mueser KT, Rosenheck RA, et al. (2014). Cardiometabolic risk in patients with first-episode schizophrenia spectrum disorders: baseline results from the RAISE-ETP study. *JAMA Psychiatry* 71, 1350–1363.

Druss BG, Zhao L, von Esenwein SA, Bona JR, Fricks L, Jenkins-Tucker S, et al. (2010). The Health and Recovery Peer (HARP) Program: a peer-led intervention to improve medical self-management for persons with serious mental illness. *Schizophrenia Research* 118, 264–270.

Galletly C, Castle DJ, Dark F, Humberstone V, Jablensky A, Killackey E, et al. (2016). Clinical practice guideline for the management of schizophrenia and related disorders. *Australian and New Zealand Journal of Psychiatry* 50, 410–472.

Goldberg RW, Dickerson F, Lucksted A, Brown CH, Weber E, Tenhula WN, et al. (2013). Living Well: an intervention to improve self-management of medical illness for individuals with serious mental illness. *Psychiatric Services* 64, 51–57.

Hamoui N, Kingsbury S, Anthone GJ, Crookes PF (2004). Surgical treatment of morbid obesity in schizophrenic patients. *Obesity Surgery* 14, 349–352.

Jarskog LF, Hamer RM, Catellier DJ, Stewart DD, LaVange L, Ray N, et al. (2013). Metformin for weight loss and metabolic control in overweight outpatients with schizophrenia and schizoaffective disorder. *American Journal of Psychiatry* 170, 1032–1040.

Liu NH, Daumit GL, Dua T, Aquila R, Charlson F, Cuijpers P, et al. (2017). Excess mortality in persons with severe mental disorders: a multilevel intervention framework and priorities for clinical practice, policy and research agendas. *World Psychiatry* 16, 30–40.

Lorig KR, Ritter P, Stewart A, Sobel DS, Brown BW Jr, Bandura A, et al. (2001). Chronic disease self-management program: 2-year health status and health care utilization outcomes. *Medical Care* 39, 1217–1223.

Ski CF, Thompson DR, Castle DJ (2016). Trialling of an optimal health programme (OHP) across chronic disease. *Trials* 17, 447.

Teasdale SB, Ward PB, Rosenbaum S, Samaras K, Stubbs B (2017). Solving a weighty problem: systematic review and meta-analysis of nutrition interventions in severe mental illness. *British Journal of Psychiatry* 210, 110–118.

Whiteman KL, Naslund JA, DiNapoli EA, Bruce ML, Bartels SJ (2016). Systematic review of integrated general medical and psychiatric self-management interventions for adults with serious mental illness. *Psychiatric Services* 67, 1213–1225.

Zheng W, Zheng Y-J, Li X-B, Tang Y-L, Wang C-Y, Xiang Y-Q, de Leon J (2016). Efficacy and safety of adjunctive aripiprazole in schizophrenia: meta-analysis of randomised controlled trials. *Journal of Clinical Psychopharmacology* 36, 628–636.

APPENDIX

Enabling and supporting patients and carers

This material is adapted and with full permission from *Psychiatric Medication Information: A Guide for Patients & Carers*, 4th Edition, Professor David Castle & Ms Nga Tran, St. Vincent's Hospital and the University of Melbourne.

We have stressed throughout this book the importance of information for patients and carers about their illness and the treatments available to them. Many organizations and pharmaceutical companies have produced such information, and there is a plethora of websites offering advice and guidance. However, many clinicians prefer to be able to direct their patients to material which they themselves have seen, and which is clearly not linked to any particular pharmaceutical product. Thus, we reproduce here sections of a booklet developed at St Vincent's Hospital in Melbourne, Australia, by David Castle and Nga Tran (senior mental health pharmacist). It has been trialled with numerous consumers and carers and refined with their input. The full pamphlet covers all the main psychiatric medications, and is available from Professor Castle (david.castle@svha.org.au).

Disclaimer

The information contained in this Appendix is not intended to be a substitute for medical care. Decisions regarding treatment are complex medical decisions requiring the independent, informed decision of an appropriate healthcare professional. Reference to any drug or substance does not imply recommendation by the authors who accept no responsibility for any clinical untoward event that may arise from following the recommendations contained herein.

Shared decision-making and medication

It is important that you and your doctor work together to make decisions about your treatment.

Remember:

- *You* are the expert about your health.
- *Your doctor* is the expert about medications and side effects.

Your doctor should provide information about all the options available for your treatment. You should ask all the questions you need to ask regarding the medications. Then you and your doctor should come to an agreement about the treatment. You need to feed back to your doctor about how you are finding the medication and discuss options if it is not going well.

> *There is a mutual obligation regarding treatments, with mutual respect and considera-*
> *tion. See it as a partnership between you and your doctor.*

Medication as part of treatment

Most of us routinely take medicine for physical illnesses. If we have a cough or cold we use decongestants, throat lozenges, or a nasal spray. When we get a headache we take an aspirin without giving it a second thought. Many people don't realize that most mental and psychological illnesses often respond to medication. So, medication taken under a doctor's supervision can play a valuable role in overcoming the symptoms of psychosis, depression, mania, and anxiety disorders. Medication may be a short-term therapy, or it may be required for a lengthy period. In some cases it may be required for many years, or even for life.

Medications are used not just to help get you well, but also to keep you well. This is the same as for many physical illnesses such as diabetes, epilepsy, and high blood pressure.

Finding the right medication

Many different drugs have proved useful in the treatment of mental disorders. Finding the right medication and dosage for each individual may require some detective work. Diagnosing the specific disorder will narrow the field of appropriate medication, and your doctor will make the final selection based on individual circumstances and your health history.

Each drug has advantages and disadvantages. Some work faster than others; some remain in the bloodstream longer. Some require several doses daily; others need to be taken only once a day. Effectiveness of medication varies with each individual. We are each unique, and so is our response to medication. Sometimes your doctor will change dosages and switch medications to find the best match between the person and the medicine.

What your doctor should know

A doctor prescribing medication must know more about the person than just the illness being treated, so a complete medical history is essential. To guard against counter-productive or dangerous drug interactions, your doctor must know what other medications (including over-the-counter drugs, herbal remedies, and other 'natural products' or substances) you are taking or have taken recently. Your doctor also needs to know about other medical problems or conditions that might affect treatment.

Risky combinations

Certain drugs should not be taken together and some drugs can be dangerous when mixed with alcohol, particular foods, or other medications. You must be thorough and honest when your doctor asks about eating habits, health history, and other drugs you are taking. Your own past experience with medication is also valuable information.

If you have been successfully treated with a specific drug in the past, that medication or one with similar properties might be preferable to an untried one. Likewise, your doctor would want to avoid prescribing a previously unsuccessful medication. Blood relatives often react to medication in a similar fashion, so experiences of family members can also be useful for the doctor to know.

Side effects and other reactions

Most people can take medications commonly used to treat mental and psychological disorders without difficulty, but sometimes there are side effects. Side effects vary with the drug but can range from minor annoyances like a dry mouth or drowsiness to more troubling reactions like irregular heartbeat. Fortunately, most side effects disappear in the first week or two of treatment. If the side effects persist, or if they interfere with normal activities, tell your doctor.

Potential side effects should be discussed before medication therapy begins. Knowing what to expect prevents unnecessary concern and alerts you to the kind of reactions that should be reported right away. Be sure to ask the doctor about the side effects you might experience with your medication (see Fig. A.1).

Scheduling and dosage

Getting the right result from medication depends on taking the right amount at the right time. Dosages and their frequency are determined by the need to ensure a consistent and steady amount of medication in the blood and by the length of time the drug remains active. If sticking to the schedule proves difficult, you

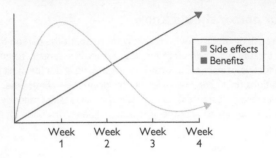

Fig. A.1 Possible side effect versus efficacy profile over time.
The new medication should help you feel better, but you may not notice the benefit straight away. Medication can take some time to start working. In the meantime, you may experience some symptoms that you are not used to. Discuss these with your doctor and within a few weeks they should settle and your treatment will be back on track.

should ask your doctor if adjustments can be made. Sometimes it is possible to change the timing of doses, although changes are not always possible. You should not deviate from the prescribed dosages unless instructed by the doctor. People who have forgotten to take their medication at some point in the day are often tempted to 'catch up' and take twice as much as prescribed at the next dose. Doubling up increases the risk of a bad reaction. The proper procedure is to take the right amount.

Believing more is better, some people increase their dosage if their symptoms are not relieved immediately or because previous symptoms have returned. Others under-medicate themselves because they fear side effects. Some people cut back or stop medication on their own because their symptoms have disappeared. Cutting dosages or stopping medications can cause symptoms to return.

Special circumstances

Using medication is more complicated for some groups of people. Pregnant women and nursing mothers, for example, must avoid certain drugs because of possible danger to the infant. If you are pregnant or planning pregnancy, tell your doctor. Young children and the elderly also need special attention. Because of their lower body weight, youngsters are generally given smaller dosages of medication than adults. Treatment of the elderly may be complicated by coexisting health problems requiring other medications, which may not mix well with the new treatment; again, lower doses are often used in the elderly.

Pregnant women and nursing mothers, for example, must avoid certain drugs because of possible danger to the infant. If you are pregnant or planning pregnancy, tell your doctor.

Tips to help you take medication regularly

To help ensure you take your medication try to:

- Take it at a set time every day.
- Link it to a regular activity such as brushing your teeth.
- Keep a simple medication diary like the one inside the front cover of this booklet or mark it on a calendar when you take it.
- Use a blister pack, sachet, or dosette® box from your pharmacy. These containers can significantly reduce the risk of dosage problems and can help you get the maximum benefit from your medication. Each dose is arranged in a separate compartment which makes it easy to check if the dose has been taken. Speak to your pharmacist for further information.
- Depots or long-acting injectable preparations can also provide a convenient alternative to taking multiple daily oral doses of certain medications.

Stopping medication requires as much care as starting it. Medications should be phased out gradually under the direct supervision of your doctor.

How long will drug therapy last?

The length of drug therapy will vary with the individual and the severity of the disorder. You are likely to need medication for at least several months. Some people may need medication for a year or longer, even for life in some cases, to keep them well.

Medication therapy generally involves a regular dosage schedule but in cases of mild or infrequent anxiety or agitation you may be prescribed 'PRN' medication to be taken at your discretion when needed.

Stopping medication requires as much care as starting it. Medications should be phased out gradually under the direct supervision of your doctor.

Strategies to deal with common side effects

Sedation

Tends to be more common on starting a new medication or when the dose is increased quickly. Starting at low doses and increasing the dose slowly can reduce the impact. Giving most of the dose at night may help, or a dose change may be required. If sedation is still troublesome, changing to a less sedating medication should be considered.

Weight gain

Can be a problem with some medications. Maintaining a healthy diet and getting plenty of exercise is recommended. Your doctor can provide appropriate support for weight management.

Dry mouth

Try taking sips of water with a bit of lemon juice in it, lemon and glycerol swabs, sucking ice, sugarless gum, etc. If none of these strategies work, ask your pharmacist about artificial saliva.

Constipation

Can be a persistent problem. A diet high in fibre, drinking plenty of water, and getting moderate exercise is recommended. Short-term use of bulk laxatives or stool softeners may be helpful.

Light-headedness

Dizziness or giddiness on standing can be a particular problem. If you get dizzy on standing, sit down, wait a little, then slowly get up again.

Nausea

Can occur in the first weeks of treatment. Taking the medication with food can help. An antinauseant medication may be needed.

Uncontrolled urination

Try to avoid drinking fluids in the evening; make sure of adequate voiding at bedtime. If the condition is troublesome, your doctor can review and prescribe particular medications to help with this problem.

Psychosis

Psychosis impairs a person's sense of reality. Psychotic symptoms vary for each person and may change over time.

Psychotic symptoms include:

- Hallucinations (e.g. hearing voices)
- Delusions (e.g. paranoia)
- Disorganized speech and behaviour.

These symptoms can occur in several mental illness disorders such as bipolar disorder, drug-induced psychosis, psychotic depression, and schizophrenia. In schizophrenia, there are also often residual 'negative' symptoms such as apathy and social withdrawal.

Psychotic episodes often occur in three phases: prodrome, acute phase, and recovery phase. The length of each phase varies between each individual and depends upon effective treatment.

What treatments are available?

Determining the best treatment options will depend on factors such as personal preference, the apparent cause of the symptoms, how severe the symptoms are, and how long they have been present. Treatment should be tailored to the individual. Individual counselling, family support, and psychosocial treatments all play important roles in the holistic care of the person with schizophrenia. Avoidance of triggers such as illegal drugs reduces the chance of relapse.

Antipsychotic medications are usually recommended as part of the treatment of psychosis to assist in recovery and prevent further relapse. There are a number of antipsychotic medications available and choice needs to be personalized to ensure the best tolerability and efficacy. Where possible, the strategy should be to start the antipsychotic at a low dose and gradually increase to minimize any side effects.

Benzodiazepines are often useful as short-term addition to the antipsychotic medication during an acute episode since they reduce agitation, tension, and anxiety and help with sleep. However, care should be taken to avoid using them for more than 4 weeks due to their addictive nature.

Antipsychotic medications

'Antipsychotics' are often effective in controlling psychotic symptoms and enable people to return to normal life. They are able to reduce distressing and disabling symptoms such as hallucinations, disorganized thinking, altered perceptions of reality, mood swings, extreme fearfulness, and severe agitation.

There are two groups of antipsychotic medications (see Table A.1).

Table A.1 Examples of antipsychotic medications

Typical or first-generation antipsychotics	Atypical or second-generation antipsychotics
Chlorpromazine	Amisulpride
Fluphenazine	Aripiprazole
Flupentixol	Asenapine
Haloperidol	Brexpiprazole
Pericyazine	Clozapine
Thioridazine	Lurasidone
Trifluoperazine	Olanzapine
Zuclopenthixol	Quetiapine
	Paliperidone
	Risperidone
	Sertindole
	Ziprasidone

All antipsychotics are effective in reducing or eliminating positive symptoms of psychotic disorders; however, the atypical or second- and third-generation antipsychotics generally have fewer side effects than the older agents, especially extrapyramidal side effects such as rigidity, persistent muscle spasm, tremors, and restlessness. Also, they may be effective in improving mood, thinking, and motivation.

How long will the antipsychotic medications take to work?

Antipsychotics begin to relieve agitation and sleep disturbances in about 1 week (see Fig. A.2). Many people see substantial improvement by the fourth to sixth week of treatment.

Antipsychotics require time to work, do not decrease or increase the dose or stop the antipsychotic without discussing with your doctor first.

How do antipsychotic medications work?

See Fig. A.2.

How long should you take this medication?

Following a first episode of psychosis, it is recommended that antipsychotic medication be continued for at least 1–2 years; this decreases the chance of becoming ill again. For individuals that have had a psychotic illness for several years or repeated psychotic episodes, antipsychotic medication should be continued indefinitely. This is similar to someone with diabetes requiring lifelong insulin.

What happens if a dose is missed?

Take it as soon as possible, as long as it is only a few hours after the usual time. Otherwise, wait until the next dose is due and take it as normal—do not try to catch up by doubling the dose.

Do they interact with other medications?

Antipsychotics can change the effect of other medications, or may be affected themselves by other medication. Always check with your doctor or pharmacist before taking other drugs, vitamins, minerals, herbal supplements, and alcohol. Always inform any doctor or dentist that you see that you are taking an antipsychotic medication.

Do antipsychotics have any unpleasant side effects?

All medicines have side effects—even the ones you can buy without a prescription at a pharmacy, supermarket, or health food store. The important thing to remember is that not everyone will have the same unwanted side effects. Side effects usually occur early in the treatment; many of them will settle down after a few weeks, when the body has adapted to the medications.

Imbalance of the brain's
natural chemicals
such as dopamine
can result in
psychotic symptoms

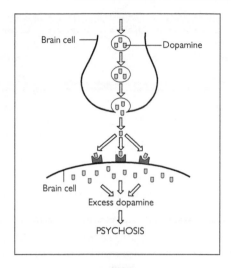

Antipsychotic
medications help
to restore the
brain's natural
chemical balance,
especially dopamine;
hence, reducing or
eliminating the
psychotic symptoms

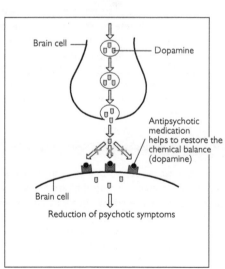

Fig. A.2 Antipsychotic medications.

Table A.2 Typical/atypical long-acting injectable antipsychotics

Typical or first-generation antipsychotics	Atypical or second-generation antipsychotics
Flupentixol decanoate	Aripiprazole extended-release injection
Fluphenazine decanoate	Olanzapine pamoate
Haloperidol decanoate	Paliperidone palmitate
Zuclopenthixol decanoate	Paliperidone 3-monthly
	Risperidone microsphere

Antipsychotic medication should not be stopped abruptly; instead, consult the prescribing doctor or pharmacist about any concerns you have.

Depots/long-acting antipsychotic injections

Depots or antipsychotic long-acting injections (LAIs) can be an important option in the context of non-adherence and can help to reduce relapse and readmission to hospital (see Table A.2). Where feasible, they should be prescribed when this is the person's preference and as part of a treatment plan in order to maintain wellness.

A test dose of oral antipsychotic may be necessary before starting LAI preparation to avoid unexpected side effects. It is important to make sure that the intended changeover is completed appropriately. For example, it is necessary to continue an oral antipsychotic for at least 3 weeks while starting risperidone LAI; while paliperidone and olanzapine LAIs, which have particular starting schedules, may not require the addition of an oral antipsychotic. Paliperidone is also available as a 3-monthly injection, but stabilization on the once-monthly is required before going onto 3-monthly.

Aripiprazole is also available in depot/LAI form. It is usually given every 4 weeks and oral antipsychotic medication should be continued for 2 weeks after the first injection.

Rarely, olanzapine depot/LAI can cause severe sedation, dizziness, weakness, altered speech, and/or increased blood pressure after the injection in some individuals so it is important to monitor for these effects for the 2–3 hours after each dose.

It may take 2–4 months for depot/LAI to achieve the desired effects so it is important to review and adjust the dose carefully.

Depots or LAI preparations can also provide a convenient alternative to multiple daily oral doses of antipsychotics.

Possible side effects of antipsychotic medications

See Table A.3.

Table A.3 Antipsychotic medication side effects and treatment

Side effects	Treatment
Muscle spasms, excessive rigidity, shaking, inner restlessness	These symptoms can be controlled with: Anticholinergic agents: benztropine, benzhexol Beta-blockers: propranolol Benzodiazepines: diazepam, clonazepam, lorazepam
Drowsiness/fatigue	This problem usually goes away with time. Use of other drugs that make you drowsy will worsen the problem. Avoid driving a car or operating machinery if drowsiness persists
Dizziness	Get up from a lying or sitting position slowly; dangle your legs over the edge of the bed for a few minutes before getting up. If dizziness persists or if you feel faint, then contact your doctor
Dry mouth	Sour candy, ice cubes, popsicles, and sugarless gum help increase saliva in your mouth; try to avoid sweet, calorie-laden beverages. Drink water and brush your teeth regularly
Blurred vision	This usually occurs at start of treatment and may last 1–2 weeks. Reading under a bright light or at a distance may help; a magnifying glass can be of temporary assistance. If the problem continues, discuss with your doctor
Constipation	Increase bulk foods in your diet, drink plenty of fluids, and exercise regularly. A bulk laxative or a stool softener helps regulate the bowels
Weight changes	Monitor your food intake. Maintain a healthy diet and try to avoid foods with high fat content. Establish a regular exercise regimen. Let your doctor know if you notice a rapid increase in your weight or waist measurement
Nausea or heartburn	If this happens, take the medication with food
Change in sexual ability/desire	Discuss with your doctor about other medications without this side effect and which may be an appropriate alternative for you

Antipsychotic medications: general precautions

- Avoid exposure to extreme heat and humidity since antipsychotics may affect your body's ability to regulate temperature changes and blood pressure.
- Antipsychotics may increase the effects of alcohol, making you more sleepy, dizzy, and lightheaded.
- Antipsychotics can impair the mental and physical abilities required for driving a car or operating machinery. Avoid these activities if you feel drowsy or slowed down.

- Do not break or crush the medication unless you have been advised to do so by your doctor or pharmacist.
- Antacids interfere with absorption of these drugs in your stomach and therefore may decrease their effect. To avoid this, take the antacid at least 2 hours before or 1 hour after taking your antipsychotic.
- Excessive use of caffeinated beverages (coffee, tea, colas, etc.) can cause anxiety, agitation, and restlessness and counteract some of the beneficial effects of your medication.
- Cigarette smoking can change the amount of antipsychotic that remains in your bloodstream, *especially clozapine, olanzapine, and haloperidol*. Inform your doctor if you make any changes to your current smoking habit.
- Do not stop antipsychotic medication suddenly as this may result in withdrawal symptoms such as nausea, dizziness, sweating, headache, sleeping problems, agitation, and tremor, and also result in the return of psychotic symptoms.
- There are differences in effectiveness and side effects between various antipsychotics; if possible, the antipsychotic with the lowest risk of side effects should be selected.
- It is essential to take *ZIPRASIDONE and LURASIDONE with food* or immediately after food to enhance the availability of these medications in your blood.
- ASENAPINE: if you are taking other medications, asenapine should be taken last. The wafer must be placed under the tongue and allow to dissolve completely. *DO NOT EAT OR DRINK FOR 10 MINUTES* because eating or drinking during this time will affect how well asenapine works.

Clozapine

What is clozapine?

Clozapine belongs to the group of medicines known as antipsychotics. This group of medicines is used mainly in the treatment of schizophrenia.

How does clozapine work?

Clozapine is used to control symptoms of schizophrenia such as hallucinations, hearing voices, and delusionary ideas. Clozapine is used in patients with schizophrenia for whom other antipsychotics have not worked or have caused severe side effects.

Things you must do while you are taking clozapine

You must have strict and regular blood tests while taking clozapine due to the rare potential problems for your blood cells. After starting on clozapine, you must have a blood test at least once a week for the first 18 weeks of treatment, thereafter at least every 4 weeks for as long as you are taking clozapine, and for 1 month after stopping the medicine.

Why is it so important to keep taking clozapine?

When taken regularly, clozapine begins to relieve agitation within the first week. Many people see substantial improvement by the fourth to sixth week of treatment. It is important to keep taking your clozapine even if you feel well as it is used not only to get you well, but also to keep you well. This is similar to someone with diabetes requiring lifelong insulin.

What happens if I miss a dose?

Take it as soon as possible, as long as it is only a few hours after the usual time. Otherwise, wait until the next dose is due and take it as normal—do not try to catch up by doubling the dose. *If you have missed taking clozapine for more than 2 days, you must contact your doctor immediately—do not start taking your regular clozapine dose again without consulting your doctor.*

What happens if I have taken too much?

Immediately contact your doctor or the National Poisons Information Service (Tel: 111 in England, Wales, and Scotland and 01 809 2166 in Northern Ireland) for advice, or go to your local Emergency Department. Do this even if there are no signs of discomfort or poisoning as you may need urgent medical attention.

Interactions with other medication

Clozapine can change the effect of other medications, or may be affected itself by other medication (see Fig A.3). Always check with your doctor or pharmacist

CLOZAPINE ALERT

Clozapine is a medication which is used to help control psychotic symptoms such as 'hearing voices'.

Take your clozapine as prescribed every day. If any of the following occurs you must inform your doctor immediately or contact SVH-PSY Triage:

- You increase or greatly reduce your smoking habit
- You commence any other medication including over-the-counter medications
- **You forget your medication for more than 48 hours**
- **If you get a sore throat, thrush or start to bruise or bleed easily**

The following **side effects** may occur:

Drowsiness, fast heart rate, excess saliva, occasional bed wetting, low blood pressure, or slow weight increase – if you experience any of these symptoms, tell your doctor.

Avoid alcohol as it may make you sleepy or dizzy. Marijuana is likely to make you ill again. Be careful with cars and machinery as you may react slower in times of danger.

You should present this card when you attend any of the following:

*Doctor   *Dentist
*Pharmacist   *Naturopath

Fig. A.3 Clozapine alert card.

before taking other drugs, vitamins, minerals, herbal supplements, and alcohol. Cigarette smoking can also change the amount of clozapine that remains in your bloodstream; inform your doctor if you make any changes to your current smoking habit.

Clozapine: general precautions

If you stop clozapine abruptly, you can experience 'cholinergic rebound' such as excessive sweating, headache, nausea, vomiting, and diarrhoea and a relapse of symptoms of psychosis.

- Tell your doctor or pharmacist as soon as possible if you do not feel well while you are taking clozapine (see Table A.4 and Table A.5).
- Clozapine may increase the effects of alcohol, making you more sleepy, dizzy, and lightheaded.
- Clozapine can impair the mental and physical abilities required for driving a car or operating machinery. Avoid these activities if you feel drowsy or slowed down.
- Excessive use of caffeinated beverages (coffee, tea, colas, etc.) can cause anxiety, agitation, and restlessness and can also increase clozapine plasma levels significantly.

Common side effects of clozapine

See Table A.4.

Rare side effects of clozapine

See Table A.5.

Always consult the prescribing doctor or your pharmacist about any concerns you have.

Clozapine should never be stopped suddenly unless your doctor tells you to.

Looking after your physical health

People with a mental illness are at increased risk for a number of medical conditions that can have a negative impact on quality of life and longevity. Also, some psychiatric medications have side effects that can increase the risk of certain medical conditions, notably heart disease. It is very important for people with a mental illness to be aware of these issues and to ensure their physical health is properly monitored and any problems appropriately treated.

Discuss these issues with your doctor and make sure you keep a record of your weight, waist measurement, and blood pressure. We also suggest you have certain blood tests done on a regular basis to monitor your physical health.

Table A.4 Clozapine side effects and treatment

Side effect	Treatment
Tiredness and drowsiness (sedation) may be troublesome	Giving most of the dose at night may help, or a dose change may be required. Contact your doctor if symptoms persist
Weight gain	Monitor your food intake. Maintain a healthy diet and try to avoid foods with high fat content. Establish a regular exercise regimen. Let your doctor know if you notice a rapid increase in your weight or waist measurement
High temperature can occur in the first couple of weeks of treatment. Sore throat, mouth ulcers, any 'flu-like' symptoms such as swollen glands, or other signs of infection	High temperature usually goes away. Nevertheless, contact your doctor to make sure there are not other causes, such as an infection, especially when the fever continues and you also have other symptoms
A fast heart beat even when you are resting is common in the first few weeks of treatment	It usually goes away. Contact your doctor if it persists or if you experience chest pain or breathlessness at the same time
Loss of bladder control, especially at night (bed wetting) can occur at any time during treatment	Changing the night dose of clozapine or limiting fluid intake before bedtime can be helpful. Contact your doctor if symptoms continue
Dizziness, light-headedness, or fainting on standing	Get up from a lying or sitting position slowly; dangle your legs over the edge of the bed for a few minutes before getting up. If dizziness persists or if you feel faint, then contact your doctor
Increased saliva production may be bothersome at night	Contact your doctor, as there are medications that can reduce/overcome this problem
Constipation can be a persistent problem	Increase bulk foods in your diet, drink plenty of fluids, and exercise regularly. A bulk laxative or a stool softener helps regulate the bowels
Nausea and vomiting can occur in the first week of treatment	If this happens, contact your doctor, as an antinauseant medication may be required

General strategies: diet and exercise

A healthy diet and regular exercise are good for not only your physical health, but also your mental health (see Box A.1). It is much better to get into a healthy habit of regular meals rather than 'fad' diets which aim to reduce weight quickly;

Table A.5 Clozapine rare side effects and treatment

Side effect	Treatment
Agranulocytosis is a blood condition where the number of white blood cells may be reduced. This is important because these white blood cells are needed to fight infection	There is no way of knowing who is at risk of developing agranulocytosis. However, with regular blood tests it can be detected early. If clozapine is stopped as soon as possible, the white blood cell numbers should return to normal. In some patients, addition of lithium (1–2 tablets) may help to restore the white cell and neutrophil numbers to normal
Myocarditis is a condition where the heart muscle is inflamed or swelling	If you develop a fast or irregular heartbeat that is present even when you are resting, together with rapid breathing, shortness of breath, chest pain, or dizziness or light-headedness, contact your doctor immediately or go to the Emergency Department at your nearest hospital. You may need to be referred to a cardiologist
Seizures or fits can occur at any stage in treatment and are often related to the dose or dose increase	Contact your doctor immediately or go to the Emergency Department at your nearest hospital when seizures occur. Your clozapine dose may need to be reduced or you may need medication to control the seizures
Diabetes, where blood sugar levels are high	Contact your doctor immediately if you experience any signs of loss of blood sugar control such as excessive thirst, dry mouth and skin, flushing, loss of appetite, or passing large amounts of urine

generally the weight stacks back on after the diet is finished and this is not good for your body.

Diet

- Try to ensure a *regular* eating pattern of three meals a day.
- *Breakfast* is a really important meal so ensure you eat breakfast every morning.
- Try to *cut out* sweets, sugar, cakes, and fizzy drinks. Junk food is not healthy: have it only as a treat, if you must, but not more than once a week.
- *Reduce* amounts of bread, pasta, potatoes, and rice. If you do eat these, use more healthy versions such as multigrain bread, sweet potatoes, and brown rice.
- *Limit* the amount of dairy you use, and consume low-fat versions of dairy produce.
- *Water is the best drink*!

Box A.1 ModiMedDiet: top 10 tips.

1. Select fruits, vegetables and nuts as a snack Have 3 serves of fruit every day Include 30g (1.5 tablespoons) of unsalted nuts daily

2. Include vegetables with every meal Eat leafy greens and tomatoes every day

3. Select whole grain breads and cereals Servings should be based on your activity levels

4. Eat legumes 3 to 4 times per week

5. Eat salmon 1 to 2 times per week

6. Eat lean red meat 3 to 4 times per week Limit serve sizes to 65--100g

7. Include 2 to 3 serves of dairy every day Select reduced fat products and natural yoghurt

8. Use olive oil as the main added fat Include 60ml (3 tablespoons) of extra virgin olive oil daily

9. Sweets for special occasions only

10. Water is the best drink

© Rachelle Opie.

Fresh fruit and vegetables are great: frozen vegetables are also good for you. Fish is excellent, especially oily fish like tuna and salmon. Red meat is ok a few times a week but must be lean (i.e. no excessive fat). Always grill or steam rather than fry. Olive oil is fantastic: pour it over salads and other foods.

It is useful to keep a food diary so you know exactly what you are eating.

Remember, alcohol has lots of carbohydrates and also stimulates appetite so can stack on weight.

Exercise

Exercise is so good for you. It helps both your body and your mind. An early morning walk in fresh air and sunlight helps get you going and also re-sets your brain's sleep–wake clock.

- Try to get into the habit of *walking* as part of other daily activities. For example, park a little distance away from your destination, or get off at the train or tram stop before your final destination, and walk the rest of the way.

- *Monitor* your daily steps: most smartphones do this for you automatically, or you can download various apps or get a pedometer. Keep a record of how many steps you do each day and then try to increase the number (aim for your 'personal best').

- You should try *exercising at least once a day* so you get a bit puffed: don't overdo it, and build up slowly week on week.
- Going to a *gym* can be good as it also allows you to socialize. Some gyms do special deals at times when they are quiet, so ask your local gym. Get a buddy to go with you for support and motivation. At least three times a week for 30–40 minutes is a good aim for the gym. Ask the gym to advise you about a schedule you can follow and ensure you know what you are doing with the various machines and weights. Again, don't overdo it, but build up slowly week on week.

Suggested metabolic monitoring

Suggested monitoring (at least 6-monthly) will vary according to the individual, their particular risk factors, and their particular medications. An example of the 'St Vincent's Metabolic Monitoring Form' successfully in use at St Vincent's Mental Health, Melbourne, is provided in this book (see Fig. 7.3 in Chapter 7): use it to monitor your own physical health and tell your doctor when your tests are due.

Monitoring should include:

- Measurement of:
  o weight
  o waist
  o blood pressure.
- Blood tests for:
  o liver function
  o kidney function
  o fasting blood sugar (for diabetes)
  o fasting blood fats ('lipid profile')
  o prolactin.

Some antipsychotic medications (e.g. amisulpride, paliperidone, and risperidone) can cause *hyperprolactinemia* (an increase in prolactin, a hormone secreted by the pituitary gland). If you are on one of these medications, you will need your prolactin level measured regularly (every 6–12 months).

Dry mouth caused by some medications use to treat psychosis and mood disorders can affect your *dental hygiene*. You should have regular check-ups with your dentist.

If you are on *lithium* you will need your thyroid hormone and lithium level measured every 6 months.

If you are on *sodium valproate* or *carbamazepine* you will need your blood count and blood levels done every 6 months.

If you are on *clozapine* you will need weekly blood tests for the first 18 weeks of treatment, and monthly thereafter, and tests of heart function (your doctor will arrange these for you).

Also, if you have any underlying *heart problems* or are on medication that might affect the heart (e.g. ziprasidone or clozapine) you should have regular tests of your heart (an ECG).

Smoking

Cigarette smoking is the primary cause of poor physical health for many people with mental illness. *Work with your doctor to try to quit smoking: your physical and mental health will be much better!* Quitting or cutting down can be very difficult since it can result in feelings of loss, sadness, and anxiety. Weight gain is also a common concern for smokers and may lead to a reluctance to quit or relapse after successful cessation; hence, good preparation and ongoing support are very important to reduce the stress associated with quitting.

The tar in cigarette smoke causes the body to break down some medications, particularly clozapine, olanzapine, and haloperidol more quickly than usual. So if you are prescribed clozapine, olanzapine, or haloperidol and are a smoker, you will probably need a higher dose to achieve the same benefit. Ordinarily this doesn't matter at all, since the dose of clozapine, olanzapine, or haloperidol you take has been tailored to suit you and takes account of your smoking (or non-smoking, as the case may be). But, if you smoke and you are considering stopping, or you have very recently stopped smoking, it is *very important* that you contact your doctor, mental health team or local pharmacist to discuss this, as your clozapine, olanzapine, or haloperidol dose may need to be adjusted.

If you have a mental illness, do not stop smoking or change your smoking habits, even if you plan to use nicotine replacement therapy, without first getting advice from a member of the healthcare team. If you have any more questions discuss these with your doctor and pharmacist.

Working with your healthcare team

Your physical health is really important, so make sure you work with your healthcare team to ensure your physical healthcare needs are being met. Take ownership of this and ensure you have regular appointments with your family doctor/general practitioner (GP). Make sure you are having regular check-ups and blood tests and keep your own record of the results: the form in this book (see Fig. 7.3) can be used for this purpose, or ask your doctor for a form or source one of the many mobile phone apps. Finally, if you are prescribed any medications, for either mental health or physical health, ask the doctor what you want to know about why they are being prescribed and the possible side effects. Once you are comfortable regarding these matters, remember to take all your medications regularly, as they cannot work properly unless you take them as prescribed.

Index